ANTI AGING

Skin Hacks & Beauty Tips to Age Gracefully

(Anti Aging Skin Care Treatments to Make You Look and Feel Younger)

Marvin Silvas

Published By Darby Connor

Marvin Silvas

All Rights Reserved

Anti Aging: Skin Hacks & Beauty Tips to Age Gracefully (Anti Aging Skin Care Treatments to Make You Look and Feel Younger)

ISBN 978-1-77485-297-2

Legal & Disclaimer

TABLE OF CONTENTS

Introduction

Everyone wants to appear younger.We are living in a culture where people place a huge value on a youthful appearance. Most of us invest a lot of energy and time - and money - to achieve this goal.We look at advertisements and are eager to buy any new product that promises to be the key to enduring youth.We scrub and exfoliate , and inject whatever the beauty and health industries have to say to us hoping that this product is the one, this ingredient that we are looking for will be the one to give us the appearance of being younger than we actually are.

I've been there.I understand how stressful costly and ineffective the quest for looking younger can be.I've seen, just like you, celebrities and other people who I know opt to undergo cosmetic surgery or chemical peels to appear younger.Even while many people scoff at the notion of injecting poison into our faces (and we all know that this is exactly the purpose of Botox is) most of us would consider it if we

1

believed it could assist in reverseing the process of aging and give us back our youthful appearance.

The downside is the truth that not all of these miraculous products and creams really work.They might temporarily boost your skin and lessen wrinkles but they're not actually helping to make your skin healthier.Expensive treatments at the salon and expensive makeup might make you feel more comfortable for a time but, at the end of the day, when you're not looking and feeling great, you'll end up sad and disappointed that you've have spent your money on some supposedly effective treatment that's in fact exactly the opposite.Instead of getting an answer to the age-defying fountain we've just exposed our body to harmful chemicals that are do not make us appear or feel younger.In reality, the reverse is true.The chemicals and substances used in these cosmetics have been accelerating the process of aging and exposing us to a myriad of ailments that can affect the quality of our lives , or even reduce them.

What's the answer? Do we simply have to surrender to the process of aging and acknowledge that we don't have any control over it? Or can we do something else that could we do in order to appear and feel better, more healthy... more youthful even?

This is where the book is in.In the pages to will follow, I'll explain the process of aging, so that you know what aging is and how it affects your body.You'll understand that treating ageing from the outside is not effective, and also the way that the additives and chemicals that are in your food items and the products you use for your beauty are harmful to your health.We'll discuss ways to combat the signs of aging on the inside with a simple and healthy habits which will alter your appearance and combat signs of aging, both external as well as external.You'll be able to harness the power of nature to attain an optimal state of health and younger appearance than before.

Chapter 1: Home Remedies For Anti-Aging

Everyone wants to appear younger and everyone desires glowing and smooth skin. This is the reason why people are making use of various odd items and products that claim to help people appear younger. The obsession to look younger has increased to the point that people are willing to eat placenta, and even apply semens of different animal species on their faces to appear younger. Additionally, many are also eager for applying harmful substances on their face and apply them to their bodies. But, it's impossible to have a flawless skin without natural ingredients and products. In this section there are many natural recipes that will aid you in achieving flawless skin in a matter of minutes. These recipes have been tested and tried, and so you can experiment with these without any hesitation.

Anti-Aging Honey Pack Honey Pack

Ingredients

2 tablespoons Organic Honey

Method

Wash your face using cold water. Pat dry using a towel clean.

Enjoy some natural, pure honey and place it in a stainless steel bowl.

Apply the honey on your face using clean hands. Massage it slowly for around two minutes.

Let it sit for approximately 20 minutes, then wash it off with cold water.

Apply toner.

Repeat this twice a week.

Benefits

Pure honey is among the greatest gifts that nature can offer. It's a wonderful moisturizer that can help reduce wrinkles.It also contains antioxidants which can help reduce the damage to skin and accelerate the process of rejuvenation.

Chapter 2: Around The World In 80 Days

Whatever you do in your travels, the one thing all nations or civilizations, cultures, civilizations and continents share is the desire to maintain the appearance of youthfulness. It doesn't matter if it's seeking out that fountain of youth or simply trying to emulate the effects of it, almost every culture on the planet offers a technique, process, or method to combat the signs of aging. In this chapter, we'll take a brief journey around the world and explore some different and effective methods to counteract the physical manifestations of ageing.

Asia:

Make a green choice with tea

Green Tea is a super drink. It packs the double benefit that it is chalk-full with antioxidants and also providing the ability to boost metabolism. Research has also proven how white tea an additional drink from china, aids skin health by protecting face from damage caused by free radicals.

In addition, it is possible to freeze tea bags and place the bags to cool your eyes for a method to combat puffiness under your eyes.

Ginger is your friend

A staple in the many meals made throughout Asia includes ginger. It is added to stir-fry, soups, tea and various other dishes, it functions as more than just a basic seasoning. It has been proven to improve circulation and help in maintaining robust immune systems. an excellent and natural approach to combat the process of aging.

You can poke yourself

Don't even think about trying this at home, folks. Acupuncture is an ancient Chinese medical method of insertion of needles into important parts of the body to reduce stress, enhance overall health, and, yes, fight the effects of aging. A positive effect of acupuncture as part of the process of preventing aging, if concentrated on for the purpose of reducing varicose veins. But, remember that the treatment is directed at reducing the size of veins and the discomfort they may cause. It is not until very rare that the veins completely disappear out of sight.

Africa:

Rooibos Tea

One drink derived from plants from Africa can be described as Rooibos tea. It is not just an amazing drink but it is also an effective way to combat some of the unpleasant consequences of aging. It is rich in antioxidants and helps fight free radicals.

Find some Gotu Kola

In South Africa, this plant is a wonder for your health. Most commonly consumed as tea it is believed that this Gotu Kola plant is said to help maintain mental clarity, and can dramatically help to reduce or prevent the appearance in varicose veins.

Australia:

Eucalyptus is your friend

To fight dry and stringy hair Try to use this Australian classic. Eucalyptus oil in shampoo will give an extra boost of nutrition and maintaining health of hair.

Europe:

Potatoes!

A popular practice used in Spain is the application of potato slices to the eyes instead of cucumber can do wonders to diminish dark circles under the eye. Because of its ability to lighten the skin, it aids in the elimination of dark circles that appear below the eyes. Therefore, next when you're reaching for the cucumbers, put it off and try potatoes.

Olive Oil

Moving out of Spain we are now heading to Italy in addition to Greece. In both countries olive oil is a useful, natural ingredient for beauty treatments. It is used by Italians for their lip conditioning olive oil is also utilized in Greece as a treatment for sunburned, dry, or other skin irritations.

Alongside the above many times, it's been claimed that olive oil can be a helpful tool in fighting gray hair when applied to your scalp, as it can help promote the growth of your hair follicles.

South America:

Get Sandy

There's no quick fix to get rid of cellulite, Brazilians have come up with some tricks to the trade. One method that is quite unique is to use sand. While it's not exactly conventional, it's been demonstrated to yield some positive results. The act of rubbing sand over areas affected by cellulite is a way to stimulate the skin and aids in diminishing this annoying age-related effect.

Avocados

Avocados can also be a well-known South American tool in fighting the process of aging. Mono-saturated fats along with the Vitamin E that is found in Avocados has been found to have a positive effect on improving the appearance of the hair and skin.

Chapter 3: What do you want in Your Life?

"There is a certain quality is required to win it, and that is the certainty of intent, the understanding of what you want as well as a burning drive be able to."Napoleon Hill. Napoleon Hill

In the beginning, you need to consider... how do would like your life to look like? Make a moment to think big and think outside of the box.

If you're still a kid with an enthralling imagination... you're in the right place! If you're an older adult, or as many are emotional jaded and damaged to the environment... you're in the right place. I urge you to be brave enough to risk it all and offer your mind the chance to be free. The ability to utilize and manage your imagination is essential ingredient to creating a more fulfilling life for you in the near future. Imagine you're a child again and everything could be possible. Take a deep breath, turn on the classic (or christmas) songs and imagine that it's Christmas morning If you could ask for anything you want in this world. what would you want? What does your ideal life be like? It's not a great life, but a dream life. If you had everything or anything. How would you like? What career path would you like to pursue? Are you employed by an company? If yes, what type? What's your position? Are you self-employed? What are you doing that is like a dream? What exactly does your ideal family appear like? Are you married? Are you a parent? Are you happy and single? What would your dream home appear like? What is it like to go through the dream home? Who's there? How do you describe the sounds, sights and smells that are in the house? Is there a celebration being held? Are you listening to music? Are you cooking up a storm inside the home? Do you really see it. What's your dream car? Imagine driving it. What would you go to if you could travel everywhere? Are you walking through one of the Venice canals that run through Italy? Are you swimming in the warm blue water of Hawaii? Perhaps enjoying some of the scents, sights delicious food and drinks at a Night market that is held located in Taipei, Taiwan? Then, what kind of impact and influence can you make to the world, if would like to? What can you do in your own life that could serve as a symbol of hope and inspire others? The most important thing is how happy and healthy would you feel in the event that you were free of limits?

Now, take a few minutes to begin this visualisation procedure. There is no limit in the world, and there is no wrong or right visions for your life's future. Also, you can give yourself the opportunity to free your mind to feel and experience the possibilities of your life.

Once you're finished you can grab your pen and paper and sketch out the kind of life you'd absolutely want to wake up every day. Be sure to include every single detail. Do you know the color of your dream car will be? Do you have an idea for the name of your dream business? If not, shut your eyes and take the details of your dream from your visualisation! Without a clear and convincing image of what it is that you would like, you won't be able to envision or experience the kind of happiness that lasts for a lifetime. If you're honest about yourself, you'll be able see your ideal life. Once you're willing to acknowledge the reality of the situation you're in Your mind will be free to explore the way to get there. would like to be and who you desire to become.

Chapter 4: Define Your Passion and Your Goals In Life to Avoid the process of aging

It's a fact that everybody ages. There's no way around that fact. Another sad fact is that everybody will be faced with declining health (in the person you love and in your loved ones) and conflict, physical impairment, and the possibility of death at one time or an additional.

These situations can cause someone to age rapidly or even prematurely. If you react negatively in these situations, you'll find yourself getting older and gaunt.

Here's how to deal with the aging process and fight the aging process:

Physical Health decline

The body's tissues break down as the person gets older. Your gums will receding and your teeth are pushed out as well as your joints and bones begin to hurt You'll begin to be weaker, it's all part of the process however, it doesn't mean you're mental capabilities are deteriorating.

You can fight aging by being more youthful. Your brain isn't deteriorating. You may notice that you're becoming distracted or forgetful at times however, it isn't a sign that you've developed dementia! You can maintain the vitality of your mind by continuing to learn and be a student of your life. You can master an entirely new language, master an entirely new skill or try an entirely new pastime, and enhance your memory with new games for memory The key word is NEW.

Learn to Elsa who is a septuagenarian in her 70s or early. She's a grandma of four and mother of five. She's also widowed. She's had to deal with a variety of issues and losses throughout her life, even declaring bankruptcy in one instancehowever, you'd be unable to tell that she's actually older until you take a glance at her ID. Many people have told her she's at least 60 years old.

Her secret? She is always on top of the changes. Her retirement could be a possibility, but she doesn't. She is still running the construction company she established many years ago, only this time, with her sons rather than her husband. As she cared for her husband who is suffering from cancer, nurses would say they appreciate her being an "millennial" grandma. This is since she has an account on her own Facebook, Instagram, and Netflix accounts. The best part is that she created them all by herself, without any help at all from her tech-savvy children and grandchildren!

So Elsa could be in her 20s however she's not letting this fact cause her to be apprehensive. She's still living her life to the fullest and discovering ways to enjoy life every single day. The loss of her husband has left an unfinished chapter in her life, however Elsa is now taking her time with determination and passion by running a company, being a volunteer for different causes, and learning Mandarin

Chinese, which is something she's always wanted to learn but had no time to do until now.

Feed your natural curiosity. It'll help you think, feel and feel younger. Don't let your brain rot. If you begin to let your mental health deteriorate the appearance and your physical health will also suffer.

Physical Disability

As we've mentioned before, physical disabilities can occur with age. If you are unable to move because of a physical limitation it's normal to be down. But, don't let the depression extend into the rest of your life. Take a look at the things that you are able to do despite your impairment. If you have vision and can use fingers, then you are able to paint, make pottery or write, or even play an instrument.

Be imaginative. Explore the possibilities. If you're having a tough to think of ideas, ask someone you love to help you. Write down everything you aren't able to do, create a second list, but this time of the things that you can DO. Examine the two lists to see what you can do to use them to your advantage. Maybe one of the items that are on the "can still do" list is a complement to (or enhances) one item from the "can't do" list. Discover the relationship between both lists and then go from there.

Conflict with family members

Family members can be a source of conflict. It's not a choice. However, what happens when it becomes a complete shouting match or even a kind of cold war? Stress from it could cause you to age prematurely particularly if you are forced to deal with that person each day.

The best way to avoid anxiety and deal with conflict with family members correctly is to pick your battles. Be aware of when you should be quiet and step away. Sure, it's tempting always be the one to say the last word but there are times when it's not worth the effort. You might have your pride intact, but you'll be left with war scars -- or , even more importantly wrinkles.

The death of a loved one

Your life can become unreal after the passing of a dear person, whether that's of a parent or child, a friend, or even a close family member. The loss of a loved one will affect your life in all aspects in your daily life.

There are a variety of coping strategies for grieving. Although grief is universal however, the experience is different to each person. People may feel isolated from this world completely for weeks and even for months. Some come back and adjust to their new lifestyle in a matter of days.

How you handle your grief could affect how you appear. Ineffective strategies for coping, such as drinking alcohol or using drugs could make you look older. In contrast dealing with grief in correctly can help you appear younger.

Here's the real-life tale: Rose is an aging widow. After a brief battle with kidney disease her husband of nearly fifty years Joe was killed. The loss of the man she loved profoundly changed Rose. She was previously a bubbly person and had a strong build. Following Joe's death she began losing the weight (to the point of appearing unhealthy and sluggish) and stopped interacting with other people, including her own children.

But, Rose kept insisting that she was "fine" when people inquired of her about her experience with Joe's absence from her life. This was her usual response until one day, one of her children forced her to look into the mirror and observe how she had changed.

It wasn't only to lose weight. Rose noticed the lines of her smile and wrinkles were getting more pronounced. Instead of laughing lines there were telltale indications of the downward twist of her mouth, as she was never smiling anymore.

The battle with her kids was the wake-up alarm Rose required. Rose realized that she had the remainder of her life to live and she should not be wasting it. She realized then that she needed to change her perspective. She needed to find her passion and reason for being when she became dating again, and was single.

It took some time it took a while, but Rose began to realize that the thing she was missing most was caring for other people. She was always selfless in her approach, and after all of her children and grandkids had grown up and gone, she didn't have anyone to care for. She admits it's simpler now that she's not being weighed down by caring duties no longer, but she longs to take charge of someone or someone or something else.

In the end, Rose took on a pet and began tending to an herb garden. It's a great, efficient method for her to deal with grief, and also find her new passion and meaning in life. These new actions and redefining her outlook have helped her appear youngerand also healthier.

The Bottom Line

What you do with life's transitions at a pace that is comfortable can make a big impact on the way you age. Many of life's snafus aren't likely to have an impression, yet certain ones -- like divorce or death that require you to think about and redefine your purpose and passion in your life. It is essential to have both because they determine the direction in which your life takes. If you do not understand the purpose behind why the reason, or the reason why the process is going, you'll get old fast.

With a positive attitude, you can cut off years off your mind as well as body. So, it's important to invest in your mental and physical well-being. If you have the right attitude you'll be able to fight the signs of ageing.

Egg Pack

Ingredients

*2 Egg whites

*1 teaspoon cream

* 1 teaspoon lemon juice

Method

A small mixing bowl, add all ingredients and mix thoroughly.

Apply the mixture above on your face, and gently massage it into your face.

Let it sit for 20 minutes.

Rinse off with cool water, then wipe your face dry using a an absorbent towel.

Apply toner.

Repeat every week twice for the best results.

Benefits

Egg whites contain anti-aging ingredients such as omega-3 acids, protein zinc, and omega-3 acids. It tightens the skin and reduces pores.

Carrots with Potato Pack

Ingredients

*1 potato

*1 carrot

* 1 teaspoon turmeric

1. 1/2 teaspoon baking powder

*Water

Method

Boil the carrot and potato in water until soft.

Slice the vegetables that you have cooked into smaller pieces.

Blend all of the above in a blender to create an even paste. Transfer the paste into an empty bowl.

Add the soda and the turmeric to the paste above and mix thoroughly. If necessary, add water.

Apply the cream gently to your face, and allow it to rest for around 20 minutes.

Rinse your face with water, then wipe your face dry using a the help of a clean towel.

Apply toner.

Repeat every week twice to get the best results.

Benefits

Carrots are a great source of Vitamin A. It is essential to produce collagen. Collagen assists in tightening the skin's muscles and stops wrinkles from developing. It is also able to help your skin to have an attractive glow. Potatoes can even out the skin tone.

Yogurt Pack

Ingredients

1 teaspoon yogurt

1 half teaspoon of pure honey

1 teaspoon lemon juice freshly squeezed

*1 vitamin E capsule (gel)

*1/2 teaspoon turmeric

Method

In a bowl, add all the ingredients, excluding the capsule. Mix thoroughly.

Make sure to puncture the capsule using an abrasive needle. Pour all the oil into the mixture. Mix thoroughly.

Apply the above mix on your face for approximately 10 minutes.

Rinse thoroughly with warm water.

Make sure your face is dry using clean towels.

Apply toner.

Repeat the process twice per week for the best results.

Benefits

Yogurt is a rich source of nutrients including vitamins, minerals and fats and more. that nourish the skin and help to keep it fresh. Lactic acid is a great ingredient to reduce pores and keep your skin tight.

Rose Water Pack

Ingredients

*3 teaspoons pure rosewater

1 teaspoon lemon juice freshly squeezed

* 1/2 teaspoon of glycerin

Method

In a bowl, combine all ingredients and mix thoroughly.

Dip the cotton ball into the mixture above, and then apply it lightly all over your face.

Don't clean your face immediately afterward.

For the best results, repeat the procedure each night.

Benefits

Rosewater is well-known for its regenerative properties. It can also increase blood circulation and decrease imperfections on the skin.

Coconut Milk Pack

Ingredients

* 1/2 cup coconut milk

*Some Cotton balls

Method

Put some cotton balls into the coconut's milk in several minutes.

Apply coconut milk with the assistance of cotton balls all over your face.

Allow it to rest over your face around 15 minutes.

Cleanse with warm water, then dry using dry towels.

Apply toner.

Repeat the process twice per week for the best results.

Benefits

Coconut is among the most effective skincare products that are naturally produced. Coconut milk is a great moisturizer for your skin, and keeps it soft and silky. It is loaded with antioxidants and nutrients to keep wrinkles at the horizon.

Banana Pack

Ingredients

1 teaspoon honey

*1 banana that is ripe

1 teaspoon rose water

1 teaspoon yogurt

Method

A large mixing bowl, peel and smash the bananas gently.

Add rose water and honey to the bowl above and mix thoroughly.

Mix yogurt with a bit of water until you have a smooth paste , free of lumps.

Apply the cream gently to your face , then let it sit for around 20 minutes.

Rinse thoroughly with cool water and wipe dry using a fresh, soft towel.

Apply toner.

Repeat the process twice per month to get the best results.

Benefits

Banana is a good in vitamins A, E as well as B. Also, it contains high amounts of iron, zinc and potassium. These nutrients are anti-aging and have anti-aging properties that help maintain an attractive and youthful appearance.

Potato Juice Pack

Ingredients

* 1 small potato

*Cotton ball

Method

Make the small mixing bowl and then finely grate the potato inside.

The potato juice can be extracted by pressing the potato to make it hard.

The juice should be strained and kept the leftovers aside. The remaining potato to make an additional face-pack.

Take a cotton ball and soak it in the juice of a potato and apply it to your face.

Dry your face for approximately 20 minutes. After that, wash it off using cool water.

Dry yourself with an untidy towel.

Apply toner.

Repeat the process twice per month.

Benefits

Potatoes are rich in nutrients, including Vitamin C that aids in the renewal of collagen. It is a great way to keep your skin elastic and tight. If you regularly use it wrinkles and fine lines could be reduced.

Papaya Pack

Ingredients

*1 small papaya that is ripe

Method

Peel and cut the papaya into smaller pieces.

Mix the pieces together in the bowl of a small dish and create an even paste. It is also possible to include a couple of drops rose water to this mix.

Apply the paste to your neck and face. Massage it gently.

Wash in lukewarm water within 15 minutes.

Cleanse yourself using fresh tissues.

Apply the toner and moisturizing.

Repeat the process twice per week to get the best results.

Benefits

Papaya is a source of a specific enzyme, known as papain. Papain is a fantastic exfoliant since it is able to remove dead skin cells and other types of skin impurities effortlessly.

Avocado Mask

Ingredients

*1 small avocado, ripe

Method

Remove the avocado pits and smash it until it forms the consistency of a paste.

Apply this paste to the face and leave it on for twenty mins.

Rinse it off by rinsing it off with warm water.

Apply toner.

Apply toner , followed by moisturizing.

Repeat every week for the best results.

Benefits

Avocados can boost your skin's radiant appearance and reduce the appearance of wrinkles and lines. Carotenoids as well as vitamin E in the fruit protect the skin from the effects of free radicals Vitamin C boosts collagen production and makes the skin smooth and firm (12).

Rosewood, Almond and Sandalwood Oil Concoction

Ingredients

1 tablespoon almond oil

*4 drops of sandalwood oil

1 tablespoon coconut oil

*2 drops of rosewood oil

Method

Combine all oils together in the glass vial. Shake the vial well.

Apply a tiny amount of oil onto your fingertips and gently rub it into your skin.

Then, let it rest overnight and clean it up in the morning.

Make sure to apply it every at night.

Benefits

The vitamins and minerals in this mix will make your skin look radiant and stay soft. It also aids in preventing wrinkles and the appearance of crow's feet.

The Almonds and Milk Package

Ingredients

*8 almonds

*Full Cream Milk

Method

The almonds should be soaked in warm milk for a night.

Blend the almonds in a blender along with the milk. Make an even paste.

Apply the cream gently to your face, and leave it on for approximately 20 minutes.

Cleanse by rinsing with cold water.

Apply the toner and moisturizing.

Repeat every week to get the best results.

Benefits

Almonds are an excellent food source for Vitamin E. Vitamin E can provide a moisturizing and rejuvenating effects on the skin, which keeps it firm and healthy. It helps slow the signs of aging , and helps keep your skin smooth and fresh.

Mashed Strawberries Pack

Ingredients

*5 ripe strawberries

Method

A large mixing bowl, mash the strawberries using a crushing.

Try to avoid lumps and create an even paste.

Put this paste on your face and allow it to rest for around 15 minutes.

Rinse yourself with tap water and wipe yourself dry using tissues.

Apply toner , followed by moisturizing.

Repeat the exercise three times per month.

Benefits

Strawberries are a great source of antioxidants. They can help keep wrinkles at low. Strawberries also have high levels of Vitamin C which improves the elasticity of skin. This pack can improve the tone of your skin and also make a few wrinkles go away.

Sugarcane Mask

Ingredients

2 tablespoons sugarcane juice

1. 1 tablespoon of curcumin

Method

A large mixing bowl, mix the juice of the sugarcane as well as turmeric powder. Mix thoroughly.

Apply the cream on your face and allow it to sit in place for 10 minutes.

Rinse your face with water, then wipe your face dry using a an absorbent towel.

Apply the toner and moisturizing.

Repeat the process 2 times per week for the best results.

Benefits

Sugarcane juice is an excellent supply of glycolic acid which gives your skin a the appearance of younger. It is also employed as an exfoliator.

Pineapple Pack

Ingredients

*2-3 slices of fresh pineapple

Method

Apply the pineapple slices to your face for approximately five minutes.

Rinse off with cold water, and repeat the rinse after 10 minutes.

Make sure your face is dry using a the help of a clean towel.

Apply the toner and moisturizing.

Repeat the exercise three times a week to get optimal results.

Benefits

Pineapple has a variety of phytochemicals as well as micronutrients that help reduce signs of ageing effectively.It can also be a great in Vitamin C which helps in collagen production.

Essential Oils Mix

Ingredients

*6 drops rose geranium oil

*6 drops of sandalwood oil

*6 drops jasmine oil

*6 drops of frankincense oil

*6 drops of neroli oil

Method

Incorporate all the oils into one small vial, shake thoroughly.

Utilizing a cotton ball place a couple of drops the oil to your face. Massage gently.

Repeat the process every night for maximum results.

Benefits

The combination of these oils can help fight wrinkles and lines. The oils are rich in omega-9 and omega-7 acids which will keep your skin looking smooth. This is an excellent moisturizing agent that can help dry, flaky skin.

Natural Concoction for the Eyes

Ingredients

*10 drops of hazelnut oil

*8 drops of carrot seed oil

*6 drops of sandalwood oil

*8 drops of chamomile oil

Method

Inside a glass container, place all the oils, one at a time and mix them thoroughly.

Place a few drops of the mix under your eyes and rub it around in an upward motion.

Sleep in the room for a night.

Repeat each night to get the optimal results.

Benefits

This cream can help reduce dark circles and crow's-feet. It can also help reduce puffiness and dryness as well.

Flower Mask

Ingredients

Six drops of olive oil

1 cup of marigold flowers

*1 cup rose petals

*1 cup of chamomile flower petals

*Water

Method

Mix all the ingredients together and make a smooth paste. Avoid lumps.

Apply the paste in a smooth manner on your face, and allow it to dry for around 20 minutes.

Rinse off the face with lukewarm water, then pat your face dry using an untidy towel.

Apply moisturizer and toner on the face.

Repeat the process every week for maximum results.

Benefits

This mix is very beneficial to your skin. It will reduce the appearance of wrinkles, fine lines and wrinkles. and makes your skin appear radiant and smooth.Apply often to keep your skin smooth, radiant and wrinkle-free skin.

Castor Oil

Ingredients

1. teaspoon Castor Oil

Method

Use a few drops the oil onto your fingertips and gently massage it on your skin.

Allow it to sit for approximately 50 minutes. If possible , let it sit overnight.

Benefits

Castor oil is a great way to reduce wrinkles and fine lines. It also helps with dry skin.

Lemon Juice

Ingredients

1 tablespoon of fresh, lemon juice

Method

Fresh lemon juice can be applied over your face. Be sure to pay focus on dark spots and age spots.

Rinse off with cool water within 20 minutes.

Apply toner , followed by moisturizing.

Repeat each day to get the maximum results.

Benefits

Lemon juice is mild bleaching agent, which can help reduce the appearance of age spots and blemishes.

(Indian Gooseberry) Amla Powder

Ingredients

Four teaspoons (Indian Gooseberry) Amla powder

*2 teaspoons honey

*3 teaspoons yogurt

*1 teaspoon of lukewarm or lukewarm water

Method

Small mixing bowl, add amla powder, yogurt, honey, and hot water. Mix thoroughly.

Smoothly all across your face.

Cleanse with water within 20 minutes.

Apply toner , followed by moisturizing.

Repeat the process once per week for the most effective results.

Benefits

Amla is high in Vitamin C and is great for hair and skin. It increases in the formation of collagen. It smooths skin and makes it elastic. When you regularly use it your skin will get firm and elastic.

Chapter 5: Changing Your Diet And Your Habits

Going Raw!

You've probably realized this after learning about the benefits to stay clear of processed foods, animal protein and cooked food.The best way to eat healthily is to eat an eating plan that is free of animal proteins and cooking.That is why you should eat raw vegan food.

What is the definition of a Raw Vegan Diet?

Veganism is the method to eat that avoids all animal products.That means you can't eat fish, meat, poultry eggs, dairy products, eggs or any other item made out of an animal.Vegans have all their calories daily from plant ingredients.

Raw diets are exactly what it seems like.People who adhere to a raw diet don't prepare the food.That means that the food they consume is not cooked.Eating this way is a good way to avoid certain foods that must be cooked before they can be consumed, for instance grains.

Combine these two concepts (veganism and raw food) together The end result is raw vegan diet.In terms of an entire diet of plant-based products that are not cooked.

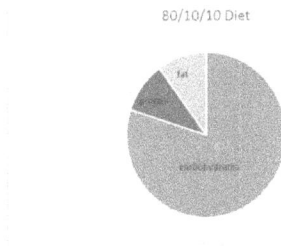

80/10/10 Diet

Knowing the 80/10/10 Diet

The 80/10/10 Diet is a type of diet introduced through the Dr. Douglas N. Graham in his book The 80/10/10 Diet.Dr. Graham was an athleticist who's been on raw food since 1978.He created the original 80/10/10 diet to aid athletes reach their peak performance.

The numbers on the diet 80/10/10 refer to the amount of calories consumed from three different categories of macronutrients.80 percent of the calories in this diet come from natural sources of carbohydrates, such as the raw fruit and vegetables.10 percent of the diet is lean vegetable protein, while the remainder is derived from healthy fats.

You can clearly see that the bulk of the calories that are consumed in the diet are from carbohydrates. This is in stark contrast to many low-carbohydrate diets available there.Contrary contrary to what many believe carbohydrates aren't the enemy.Processed sugars - like table sugar are not healthy for you.The same is true for other types of sugar that are that are used in processed food such as health hazards like high-fructose corn syrup as well as corn sugar.Eating food items with a high amount of processed sugars is certainly not a great idea.However the sugars that are present in fruit aren't processed.Fruits are full of fibers that help the body to digest the sugars they contain without affecting blood sugar levels.

Most vegetable leaves that are green and leafy are extremely low in calories.For example, you'd need to consume about 20 head of romaine leaf for 2 000 calories.Obviously the green leafy vegetables are extremely nutritious and are essential to the 80/10/10 diet. However, it's just not practical to consume enough green veggies each day to achieve a recommended daily calorie intake of around 2200 calories.That implies that a substantial portion of the calories consumed by those who adhere to the 80/10/10 diet is derived from fruits.

You may be asking questions about nutrition.How can you make sure you are getting sufficient nutrients that you currently get from animal proteins grains, dairy, and other sources even if you're not eating these foods?

How to get Nutrients from Raw Diets? Raw Diet

Some critics of raw veganism argue that it is impossible to obtain all the essential nutrients that we require by the Raw vegan diet.When people first begin eating a raw vegan diet they typically ask "How do we get the nutrients we've been taught to be obtained the animals?"

Consuming a raw vegan diet means you will need to be aware of the minerals and vitamins in the food items and vegetables in order to ensure that you're getting the right nutrition.For instance, let's take a take a look at calcium.Most guidelines state that we should consume around 1,000 milligrams calcium every day. The pharmaceutical and dairy industry has us believing that we should depend on dairy products like milk for calcium.Nowadays we know that dairy products aren't an excellent source of calcium and, in reality as with the other products of animals causes calcium deficiency. Dark leafy greens, such as mustard, spinach, kale greens , and collard greens are all great sources of calcium. Moreover, several other vegetables and fruits also contain calcium.

The best way to ensure you're getting enough nutrients is eating a diverse assortment of fruit and vegetables.Often the color of a plant or fruit is a sign what nutrients contains.If you ensure that you include yellow, green fruits, red, and oranges in your daily meals and you'll be sure that you're receiving the right amount of nutrients and minerals.To help you gain a greater knowledge about this issue, below are a few advantages to health outlined through the colour of a particular fruit or vegetable:

Yellow and Orange and orange vegetables are abundant in bioflavonoids, antioxidants, and carotenoids, aswell with potassium, and Vitamin A.Eating both orange and yellow fruits and vegetables like sweet potatoes, carrots yellow peppers, oranges, butternut squash and more helps improve eyesight, improve blood pressure, and strengthen the immune system.

Red fruit and vegetables are an excellent source in Vitamins A and C along with lycopene and quercetin.A diet that is rich in red fruits and veggies like raspberries, cherries, apples tomatoes, red onions and tomatoes helps prevent lung, cervical and prostate cancers, decrease bad cholesterol, boost joint health , and improve digestion.

Green: We all know that leafy green vegetables are a great source of calcium.Green fruits and vegetables like broccoli, arugula, apples , and avocados are excellent sources of folate, chlorophyll, lutein and beta-carotene. They also reduce cancer risk and improve digestion.

I strongly suggest that you utilize various websites or apps to track your diet and health information. I usually use https://cronometer.com/ to find out what every single fruit and vegetable contains in it.

What is a Raw Vegan to consume in a day?

In this case it might be beneficial to consider what you can be eating on the course of a typical day when you follow the raw vegan diet.If you're just beginning to learn about this type of diet it may be hard to figure out how you can make a vegan diet work for you.

Breakfast

When you first get to get up, sip an enormous glass of water.This will allow you to refresh your body after going for a long time without water.A many raw vegans prepare made juices or smoothies to serve for breakfast.A smoothie is ideal to fill you up and gain energy to get through the day.If you're worried about staying full, a drink is the best option since it is made with fresh fruits and vegetables which means you'll receive the right amount of fiber that will keep you full for.

The beauty of smoothies is that it is possible to put whatever you like into it.As raw vegans is essential that you consume enough dark leafy greens. Therefore, try including certain kinds of them in your smoothie.You will be able to maximize the quantity of nutrients you absorb by eating those foods that contain the most amount and variety of nutrients. This will be a breeze those who eat plenty of fruit and leafy greens since they are among the most nutritionally high-nutrient food items.

Green leafy vegetables are packed with a variety of vital nutrients like omega 3 as well as calcium and vitamin C, among others. They'll make your smoothie green. However, when you add fruit, you'll end up with tasty drinks that supply you with calcium, protein, and lots of nutrients and minerals.Using avocados or bananas can make your smoothie have a lovely smooth texture.You could also freeze certain fruits for a rich, cold smoothie.Some ideas for combinations include mangos and bananas in a spinach smoothie or kale mixed with apples, celery, and banana.Experiment to discover which combination you like best!

If you do not want to drink smoothies and prefer eating the whole fruit.Some raw vegans prefer to eat only one kind of fruit with their meals and others prefer to keep several varieties. variety.They must consume foods that satisfy you, and eat enough to keep your body energized.

Lunch

A lot of raw vegans consume fruit to eat lunch as well.Remember that if you're adhering to the 80/10/10 diet, the most of your calories are likely to be derived from fruit.You can enjoy a meal of just one type of fruit or several varieties. variety.One important thing to remember when you eat in this way is to consume whatever is in season.If nectarines and peaches are in the season, your lunch might include ten mature peaches.The advantage of whole fruits is that they're extremely portable, which means that even during an extremely busy day, you can take them along and take them with you on the move.

If you are looking for a more savory lunch, there are plenty of delicious options.You can cut vegetables and wrap in nori to create vegan rolls.You can prepare a large salad and serve it with a tasty dressing.The only limitations are your personal preferences and the amount of preparation you'd like to make prior to when eating.

Dinner

If you want to eat a basic dinner it is possible to start with some fruits and prepare a huge salad.Remember that there aren't too many calories in the greens, so it is important to consume plenty of them.You may have two bunches of lettuce (or equivalent quantities of kale, spinach, as well as mixed baby greens) and you can then add a variety of other vegetables.Some options to consider include bell peppers that are multi-colored as well as cucumbers, carrots and tomatoes.It's an excellent idea to add healthy fats and consider adding seeds or nuts or avocado slices.You can make dressing with the blended veggies as well.One way to do this is by mixing ginger and carrots for the dressing, or adding tomatoes and basil.

If you'd rather making your own noodles, make zucchini noodles by using spiral cutter.You can then top them with delicious tomato sauce.You could also make vegan tacos by using lettuce wraps to make shells. shells.The possibilities are limitless.

Snacks

Sliced vegetables and fruits make excellent snacks.You can carry them around with youand even make a dip sauce to accompany them.If you're looking for something different Try stuffing the ripe dates in raw nut butter? Don't be scared to be creative.It's essential to diversify your food choices - this will ensure you're getting many different nutrients and will also assist in avoiding boredom.There numerous fantastic alternatives available!

Don't forget to drink plenty of fluids throughout the day.Staying hydrated will aid in your digestion as well as keep your skin looking healthy and radiant.

Protein as well as Muscle Mass

We've already spoken a on the significance of consuming sufficient protein in your diet.You are aware how dark-colored greens can be a great source of protein, and so do nuts as well as seeds.All foods and vegetables have some form of protein, but how do you ensure that you're receiving enough?

(Again, I suggest you use https://cronometer.com/ or some other nutrition information you can find to track your nutrition)

It is possible to calculate how much protein you require by weighing yourself - the recommended amount for a person who is sedentary can be .36 grams of protein for every pound body weight that is .8 grams of protein for every kilogram body weight.Protein helps to protect bone density and assist in the repair of muscles tissues.Getting the right nutrition is just one aspect of the picture.It's essential to exercise well.One among the more essential types of exercise (at all ages!) is lifting weights.

Why is weight-training so vital? For starters the body tends to build muscle slower when we age.Keeping your muscles healthy and strong will help you look and feel younger.Having strong muscles means it is less likely that you'll injure yourself.Your muscles and bones are a team that aid your body.Weight training helps protect your bones.As we age we are prone to losing the density of our bones and muscles and this is the reason why fractured bones are so prevalent in those who are elderly.This is particularly true for post-menopausal women who lose a little less than 2% of their bone mass each year following menopausal symptoms. The greater the muscle mass you possess the greater chance it is to aid in increasing the overall calories burned all the time and make your skin looking younger.

Training for weights can improve or even eliminate some of the ailments that we experience as we age.For instance, a study conducted by the Center for Disease Control showed that people suffering from arthritis saw an increase of 43% in discomfort after a weight-training program during six weeks.Weight training helps strengthen the heart and boosts the overall health of your cardiovascular system, which is something that many of us are concerned regarding as we age.It will also help keep blood sugar levels in check and improve sleep at night.

One of the main benefits of training with weights is that it can make you feel more youthful and happier.Studies have proven that exercise can reduce depression.This could be due to a biochemical shift that takes place within the brain during exercise.It could happen due to the fact we generally be happier overall when we feel more healthy and more powerful. Most likely, it's the combination of both the above things.Being physically active can have repercussions that go beyond the physical benefits of the workouts you're doing.Being more physically active can aid in staying alert and active in your mind and emotionally and mentally well.Weight training and exercising are essential components of living a healthy raw vegan lifestyle and a healthy one all around.

Chapter 6: Your Diet And Aging

While establishing healthy, well-balanced practices is a great way to live longer however, it is crucial to keep in mind the ways in which a healthy diet can be beneficial to you. From your brain to your bones, the food we consume ends in playing a major role in the way we get older. When we eat the right food, will help improve our bodies and minds healthier and better able to endure longer and longer without causing accidents and a sagging skin. Here's a list which are suggested to slow the process of aging within our bodies:

Fruits and vegetables

A major component of our food regimen and one that is often overlooked. The vibrant fruits and vegetables contain antioxidants. You've likely heard of this before, but what is an antioxidant? Antioxidants are chemical substances that are found in foods and supplements that have the capability of reducing the effects of oxidation on tissue. It is important to keep in mind that this process, while harmful to body and the other tissue is normal. There is no way to stop it, however you can reduce the damage by eating healthy foods like fruits and vegetables.

When we eat foods that contain Vitamin C, Zinc and Beta-carotene, we are able to preserve our vision by preventing the development of ocular degeneration, which is one of the main causes of blindness among older adults. The leafy greens like Kale, spinach, and colourful produce like cantaloupe, oranges and corn are loaded with the three essential antioxidants.

If you're a fan of wine you'll be delighted to know that an antioxidant found in red grapes in wine, resveratrol, is an amazing antioxidant that helps protect your body from the damage linked to heart disease and cancer by reducing inflammation and stopping the oxidation process of LDL cholesterol. To summarize If you'd like to enjoy the pleasure of a glasses of wine occasionally, absolutely take it.

Fish

Fish is extremely rich in Omega-3 fatty acids, which provide amazing anti-aging benefits. Omega-3's aren't only essential to our health, but can also aid our bodies in decreasing cholesterol levels that can increase the risk of developing heart disease. Two Omega-3 acids in particular (EPA as well as DHA) can help improve the condition of your joints. They can also reduce joint stiffness. This will make you feel younger. In addition, certain Omega-3 acids may moderately boost your mood and can interact with certain antidepressants to increase their effects. It's recommended to seek out Omega-3's through natural foods, however supplements are also fine, however the absorption rate is higher when you get it through natural resources. A few of the kinds of fish that have the highest levels in Omega-3 fats include mackerel, herring and anchovies as well as salmon (try to go for wild-caught whenever you can) as well as tuna and trout.

Dairies

I've been following a thread on food health in which dairy products are being criticized due to their excessive levels of fats hormones, and the adverse effects they have on certain individuals' digestive system. I'm not certain why this dairy-war is gaining so popularity, but I'm worried about it as the majority of dairy products are great. Vitamin D and calcium that are found in cheese, milk and yogurt play an important part in keeping the strength of our bones and help prevent osteoporosis. Selecting dairy products that are low in fat will aid in keeping your cholesterol levels in check, which will lower the chance of suffering from stroke, heart disease and other.

If you are suffering from a an actual lactose intolerance (another term that I hear thrown around so often) it is possible to find dairy products that are lactose free however they are filled with vitamin D and calcium.

Nuts

Every kind of nut (as as long as they're not salted) are incredibly anti-aging. Cashews, walnuts, almonds and pecans are all great, when eaten consumed on their own or as a supplement to other foods in this list like yogurts, salads or salads. Walnuts are high in Omega-3 acids as well as being high in monounsaturated fats (one of the "good" healthy fats) that can help to improve your heart's health. In general, a serving of 10 to 15 nuts that are not salted daily will provide amazing health benefits without adding a lot in calories into your daily caloric consumption.

Tea

The tea itself is loaded with antioxidants. If you want to make the effort choose green tea as well as black tea. Black and green teas contain 10 times the antioxidants present in the fruits and vegetables. Black tea and green tea are both derived of the same plant. Camellia Sinesis, which is abundant in polyphenols, an antioxidant which helps to detoxify cells in our skin as well as other tissues. The plant also has plenty of epicatechins as well as catechins. Two of the best antioxidants that the body needs are catechins and epicatechins because they aid in reducing toxins that are that are linked to cancer and atherosclerosis.

Berries

The berries are well-known for their anti-aging benefits as they are loaded with flavonoids which are powerful antioxidants that help protect your body from aging and free radicals. The best part of berries is they are a variety of ways to consume them, blend them into your cereal or yogurt then freeze them before blending with delicious smoothies or take them on their own fresh or dried! The berries are available all year long and relatively inexpensive. It is worth purchasing them in bulk and freeze them in the event of need.

Research suggests that a cup of mixed fruits every day can provide all the antioxidants you require within a day. However, I would suggest that you obtain antioxidants from a variety of food sources and supplements since it is more easy for you body absorb them.

Foods to stay clear of

You'll be surprised by the fact that it is very likely eating a diet that is delaying you or hindering your fighting against aging. What you put in your mouth will determine how quickly you get older and how quickly the signs of aging will appear within your body. When you eat foods that aren't of high quality like refined sugars and simple carbohydrates, you'll end up damaging collagen on your skin, making appearance tired and aged over time.

Foods such as Trans fats are also shown to trigger constipation and inflammation that can impact the well-being of your digestive, circulatory and nervous system by keeping toxins out of your kidneys, GI tract and blood.

It is also an ideal idea to reduce the amount of deep-fried and battered foods you consume. Anything that's been deep and fried may cause inflammation throughout your body. Be cautious about food items that contain Trans fats as they increase LDL cholesterol and decrease good cholesterol. Be sure to look over the labels of your food for any warning signs that pop up. If you're not sure, it's best to stay clear on it.

Chapter 7: The Anti-Aging Mindset

If you believed that preventing aging is just about eating certain foods that are nutritious and consuming some magical cures You may be disappointed. There is no magic food or remedy that can reduce the effects of an your unhealthy, harmful lifestyle that you may have led for a long time. It's a bit more complex as that.There are, naturally very beneficial food items and treatments that can bring you to the top of your game. They are described in the next chapters. However, you must to rid yourself of any unhealthy habits and you must start now.

Don't make the mistake of expecting dramatic transformations that will happen immediately or even a few weeks later after you've made the decision to alter your routine. It requires time. It requires persistence. It requires some difficult choices to be re-evaluated and repeated. You must think about the long term, as the effects will not be apparent for months, or perhaps for years. You'll be unsure of what you would be like if you had not taken that step. It's not easy to take at times and it's incredibly easy to give up and then not do it again, but it's not as difficult as it appears. While there aren't ways to avoid it, there are tried and tested methods to save yourself from disappointment and allow you get younger, instead of becoming older, at the very least for a few years.

It is crucial to be aware of exactly what you're doing and why you're doing it. Be aware of the risks, as they're as high as they could be. Imagine an active and healthy 50 year old, or a 60-year old, or even an 80-year old you've seen. Imagine an individual who's opposite of them poor, sick or depressed. Imagine the real individuals you have met is a fantastic way to envision your own future prospects. Imagine yourself being around two decades older the person you are as you read this. It will be the same face, familiar to you with some wrinkles. The appearance of your skin could change and your hair may turn increasingly or lesser gray. Which is something you are able to hide. However, there's more. Your silhouette could change more that your appearance. Your back may be bent just a bit. It could also be a bit more. Your movement, overall energy and the sparkle in your eyes are all dependent on what you're doing to improve your health now. It can be challenging to keep all of this in your mind at all times. So prior to beginning to build your muscles -- and soon discover the reasons to build up your muscles to fight the aging process, you'll have to focus on your mindset.

As you are aware, there are two main mentalities: the fixed and the growth mentality. Growth mindsets are focused on personal development and growth. The fixed-minded on the other hand is focused on inherent traits. This isn't a book about mental states however, let's take an examination of how different mental models can influence your thinking about aging, and then to think about the topic of the book, anti-aging.

Someone with a fixed mentality tends to view the aging process as a hard biological fact. As time passes, you become older. Inevitably. It's inevitable. There's no way to stop it. Your fitness level or health, the level of your functional capacity--all are based on the age you are at and your genetics. And you can't change your genes. It is either your nature to be attractive healthy, fit and healthy and fit, or you aren't as. You might be blessed with inherited a "skinny gene" or a "fat gene." Again, there's nothing you can do about it, other than to relax with a slice of cake. And then, one day, you might experience an attack on your heart or stroke, or be diagnosed with diabetes. It isn't your fault in any way. It's all down to the genes. A fixed mentality urges you to take advantage of your retirement savings to take some time off. You take a lot of rest like you're in your 90s rather than your sixty-six. The clock ticks by as you lie on your couch while watching TV and eating a few more calories than you may burn off while getting older and then waiting to die for a long time.

It was quite a shocking image, wasn't it? I'm confident that you're most likely to are blessed with good genes. The majority of human beings do. We've become the people we are today because of the long evolution process. You were created to become an athlete. You're blessed with a brilliant mind. You can utilize your mind as well as your body in a manner that allows you to stay young beautiful, healthy, and attractive longer than every other creature on earth. However, it is important to be a responsible adult. You are responsible not to compromise the potential of this amazing opportunity through sitting on your sofa eating unhealthy food and watching TV.

We'll return to our mindsets. In contrast to the fixed mind is the growth mentality. If you are in the growing mindset you're the one in charge. It's your responsibility to maximize your potential genetically and improve it. This is what you've inherited as a potential. Everything else rests on your shoulders. It is important to note that the majority of people do not achieve their maximum potential, never push themselves to their limits, never living fully. It's much easier that approach. However, you are heading in a different direction right now. The right mindset can allow you to expand. When you are in a growth mindset there are many possibilities that you could ever imagine. With this type of mentality, you could become functionally older than you currently are and stay young for whenever you want to. You exercise enjoying yourself, cognizant of how much progress that you are making. When you are in the right frame of mind you start to enjoy the hard work. When you are in the right frame of mind you are more inclined to eat healthy. You are happy by avoiding junk food and drinks. It's a fact that you'll live longer and longer. Your life is in your own hands, and your limits remain waiting to be seen. With a fixed mentality the people think their hands are tied. only thing they can do is watch the devastation of their bodies and spirits in silence. The destruction is happening slowly and continuously, at the level of the cell, until it becomes apparent, eventually, they age quickly, and eventually pass away. The method of thinking and the belief of being able to stop decline is essential to stop the degenerative process in the first place. You only must make a clear choice to fight ageing, and choose to live instead of decline, and read the rest of the book and you'll be able to figure out what to do in the future.

Chapter 8: Men's Skin Care

Men's skin care could be perceived by certain men as a new topic. It would have been unfamiliar a few years ago. In reality, a rising amount of men understand the importance of skincare for men (and that's why you see areas with male-specific skincare products as well). "Man skincare" is very similar to products for women, however the male's skin is different from the female skin.

"Man skin care" also begins with cleansing. Cleansing helps to prevent the clogging of pores and also helps remove dirt and pollutants off your skin. The natural greasy character for male skin is what makes it an essential part of the male skincare process. It is essential to wash your face at least once a day, but it is better the cleaning is completed on a every day.

Shaving 'Man Skin Care can be a bit of a flurry. Shaving cream, solution, aftershave and products include among the top important male skin care products. The essential'man's skin includes a variety of shaving products and equipment. The most crucial factor to consider when choosing shaving products must be the type of skin (because the amount of oiliness differs from person to).

Alcohol-based aftershaves should be avoided. The proper'man's skin requires use of high-quality blades. The turning-head blades below are selected because they have been known to reduce cuts. In addition to the gear and products are also essential to use the right ones.

Male skin tends to be oilier and heavier due to more pores and sebaceous glands that are active. However, because of the frequent exfoliation, your skin can be dry without problems. Therefore, lotions are an integral part of skincare. The moisturizing gel or product should be used following shaving. Some shaving foams/solutions contain an inbuilt moisture-enhancing effect. Creams should be gently massaged using upward strokes.

They must be applied gently within the sensation.

Utilizing a sunscreen is an essential measure for men's skin however, a man's face is more susceptible to developing skin cancer as a result of the ultraviolet radiation. It is essential to apply an item that provides moisturizing effects and sunscreen.

Another option for man's skincare is to use male-specific skincare products that contain organic ingredients like aloe Vera sea salt, grapes and aloe Vera oil that fights off bacteria. e.g. Teatree, teatree, etc. provide an great solutions for male skin care.

Male skincare is not as difficult for a lot of men believe. To supply you with a clean and healthy skin in the near and future, you just need to spend just a few minutes every throughout the day.

The necessity of caring for the Skin

"Packaging is just as important as the present itself" is a statement that many of the current manufacturing companies adhere to with great care. The same is true for you, too. Your exterior self, i.e.. your face is as crucial as your home inside. Many people are aware of the importance of taking care of their skin. This is among the reasons you can see several skincare products available on the market. The majority of skincare products perform very well. It is common to think of with skincare a good appearance. But the benefits go beyond this. There are numerous benefits associated with glowing and balanced skin

First of all, it has an effect on your self. It makes you feel energetic and fresh. You'll feel more productive to complete your tasks and are more prepared to tackle more tasks you need to complete. In addition, the flavor enhances every day life and your enjoyment. A healthier, more youthful skin contributes to creating confidence. Sure, you can claim all the credit for being able to achieve this (however be sure to take a moment to consider skin care products)

Furthermore, this flow of positive energy is experienced by others around you and you notice that they're more friendly to you. You will gain greater value from people around you. You will be more attentive when they answer your inquiries. They also experience the enthusiasm that you radiate. They are enthralled by dealing with you and also with you. Yes , it does work. People might be interested in asking you regarding the skincare products you use (you may or might not display the essential skin care products for them). A healthy, glowing skin is an important factor in creating a relaxing and relaxing environment for you.

However the opposite, neglect or naivety on this shirt can make you appear unattractive as well as boring. You'll be lively, but find yourself feeling boring. Your performance at work is diminished. Some of the people you meet could be hostile. It could result in you getting older and starting in later.

This is why the importance of skincare can't be undervalued. But, it's not very simple.

There's no doubt that there are a variety of products for your skin and you'll be able to choose those that are the most efficient. The information on the categories below can aid you in identifying them as well as there are many methods by which skincare products are identified and can be used to create a variety.

Another option is to classify skin care products according to their usage, for example.. There are creams as well as skincare products that help exfoliate as well as cleanser, toners, and cleansers.

* You will also have skincare products to treat various skin issues, i.e.. skincare items for acne facial products for stretch marks skincare products to fight wrinkles, etc.

Another category is based upon the components , for instance. cosmetic skincare products organic skincare products, chemical skincare items.

Skin care products aren't your only option for skincare. You also need to incorporate some basic ways to maintain your skin that you can apply to your daily routine (like we'll discuss in our other article about personal skincare).

An excellent anti-aging strategy: Make sure you get enough sleep

Can you get sleep? If you're currently trying find a solution to aging that could work ensure that you have enough rest during the process. It is a fact that as the years go by, that your body will continue to begin to age. However, the amount of aging you experience in your appearance and health could be controlled to a certain extent. Whatever option you decide to explore to reduce your signs of ageing, and improving your overall health, be sure that sleep is a part of your plan.

Sleep is essential.

Sleeping is the body's method to heal and increase. Your body makes use of your health to boost, grow to heal cells and to treat your health issues in the event that you are sleeping. Therefore, it is crucial in the process of anti-aging to take into consideration whether you have enough sleep so that your body can take the necessary steps in order to keep your skin's appearance and your overall health.

How Much Would You Earn?

Doctors have stated that people require at minimum eight hours of rest every night. Because every person is unique and has different needs, the body of a person may require more or less. The best way to determine whether you're sleeping enough is simple. Do you wake up each early morning feeling rejuvenated? Do you start your day dreaming about how exhausted and need to be able to sleep for a few more hours? In the absence of enough rest the body will not be able to perform the things it's required to accomplish. Therefore, you should look for improvements in your sleep. Here are some tips that can help you get to sleep quicker.

Beware of eating food if not eating a large meal at least 2 hours prior to going to the time you go to bed, as they increase the blood sugar levels and help you stay hydrated.

Pay attention to white noise that could be regular or even recordings of peace. Resuming a meditation before bed can help you sleep well.

Don't be a TV viewer. It stimulates your brain. is responsible for engaged and informed, is stimulated by TV. You can also find a relaxing exercise that you can complete.

It is vital to get enough sleep for those who are using anti-aging techniques or just want to boost their general health. Learn what it could help you by going to go to bed earlier and getting the sleep that your body requires. This could be the perfect complement to other strategies to fight aging as well.

Chapter 9: 100% natural recipes for treating skin infections and fighting against aging

DIY Aloe Vera Scrub with olive oil

This recipe is great to exfoliate. Cell turnover is an important benefit of making this recipe. It also increases your collagen production.

One tablespoon Aloe Gel

1 tablespoon extra olive oil

1/4 cup brown sugar

Mix all the ingredients and apply the mixture on your face. massage it gently in an upward motion. Apply the mixture for about 3-5 minutes, then wash off with water, and dry your face.

The secret to this recipe lies in the brown sugar, which aids in exfoliating dead skin. Olive oil and Aloe are rich in healing nutrients.

DIY Aloe Vera Face Mask with rose water

Before you begin the process of making this mask it is essential to cleanse your skin from any cosmetics creams, and other products. It is recommended to shower with steam.

1 tbsp. aloe gel

A pinch of turmeric powder

1 tbsp. raw honey

1 tbsp. milk

A couple of drops of rose water

Mix the ingredients, then apply the mixture to your neck and face. let it sit for 20 mins, then rinse it away and pat dry it with a the use of a towel clean. Repeat the application at least every week.

DIY Aloe Vera Mask with powdered sea green

Combine 1 tablespoon of powdered seagreen with 1 Tbsp. of Aloe Gel. Apply it to the face and let it sit in for about 10 minutes. Repeat the process every week. If you're not aware that seaweed powder increases circulation of blood, helps detoxify the body, removing impurities and softening your skin.

DIY Aloe Vera Mask with egg yolk

Mix 1TBSP. of Aloe Vera gel with 1 egg yolk and 1 teaspoon olive oil. Apply it to the face and neck for about 20 mins. I tried it , and it appeared as if I've been given a shot of Botox. Awesome!

Made at home Aloe Vera Mask with grapes

Combine 1/2 cup grapes with 1erra. consisting of Aloe Vera gel as well as 1 tablespoon. of honey in raw form. apply it to your skin for 20 mins. Repeat the procedure once every week.

Aloe Vera is among the most potent natural anti-wrinkle treatments available on Earth. It stimulates collagen production and protects the collagen that is already present.

Homemade toner using Honey and Cucumber

Puree one cucumber in a blender , then drain and then collect the juice. Add 2 teaspoons of honey to the juice, and mix the composition. Then , put the mixture into an e-liquid bottle and place it to your neck and face with an abacus pad. Then, store the mixture in the refrigerator for a week.

Home-made toner using Honey and Apple

Blend in the blender 1 cored and peeled apple along with 1erra. of honey. The mix must be smooth. Apply it to your face for 15 minutes. Then wash it off.

Homemade Face Scrub using Honey and Oats

Mix 1 tbsp. honey, 1 tbsp. almonds, 2 tbsp. dry oatmeal, yogurt or lemon juice to make an incredible facial scrub. Rub it lightly on your face and allow it to dry for 30 minutes before washing with warm water.

Homemade Face Mask made with Honey and Nutmeg

This mask is a great solution for healing acne scars. It's extremely effective for anti-inflammatory purposes, to prevent skin infections, heal the scars and cleansing your skin thoroughly.

1 tbsp. honey

1 teaspoon ground Nutmeg

Mix the honey and Nutmeg and apply it on your face. It should be in the area of your face where you have acne. Allow it to sit for 30 minutes , and then rinse it off.

Homemade mask using cocoa and honey

This mask is extremely beneficial to revive dull skin and regenerating it. It's a fantastic treatment for aging skin. Although it's difficult to imagine, it's true that chocolate is loaded with antioxidants that nourish your skin and make it look radiant and soft.

1 tbsp. honey

1 teaspoon of cocoa powder

Mix the honey and cocoa powder. Spread the mixture on your neck and face and allow it to work for about 30 minutes. After that, wash it off.

Homemade scrub using sugar and olive oil for your body

One cup sugar(brown or white)

1/4 cup olive oil

It is also possible to include the essential oils and herbs, or honey. This scrub is fantastic in your personal care, specifically for moisturizing and exfoliating your legs and arms.

A homemade olive oil scrub for the face

1 teaspoon olive oil

2 teaspoons baking soda.

Blend the ingredient until have the consistency of a paste. You can also add lemon juice or honey into the mix. Apply it to your face to remove dead skin cells for about 10 minutes, then cleanse it off with warm water.

Your skin will get the most incredible benefits of emollients and emollients from this scrub. It is believed that olive oil can be described as considered to be the Liquid Gold for your skin. It is a natural source of antioxidants that combat free radicals that are harmful and can cause aging of your cells.

Made at home Avocado face mask using lemon juice for normal skin

This recipe is fantastic to moisturize your skin and eliminating dead cells.

2 tbsp. mashed avocado

1 tsp. fresh orange juice

1 tsp. lemon juice

Mash the avocado, then mix in the orange juice and lemon juice. Mix it up until you've got a smooth and creamy paste. Apply it to your skin for around 20 mins and afterwards wash it off using lukewarm water. It is recommended to use it at least once per week.

Made at home Face Mask with green tea for normal skin

This recipe is hydrating and helps maintain an equilibrium between the fatty acids and water within the skin. It stops the aging process of cells.

2 tbsp. mashed avocado

1 tsp. yogurt

1/2 tsp. Green tea that has been blanched cuts

Mash the avocado, and then mix in green tea. Grrate the tea to ensure it turns into a powder. put it into a fine strainer , and then boil it. Add the yogurt. Apply it to the skin and leave it for about 15 mins and then wash off using lukewarm water. Make use of this mask every week.

Avocado face mask at home made with olive oil to treat dry skin.

This mask softens and moisturizes skin, cleanses dead cells, and combats wrinkles.

1 tbsp. mashed avocado

1 tbsp. of mashed banana

1 tsp. olive oil

1 tsp. fresh orange juice

Mash the avocado, and then add olive oil, orange juice, and the banana. Mix all the ingredients until you have a smooth and even paste. Apply it to your skin , avoiding the eye area, and leave it sit for 15 minutes. Then, wash it off using lukewarm water. The mask can be applied at least once per week.

Face mask made from avocados that is homemade using Honey and Almond Oil for dry skin.

This mask assists in protecting our skin from damage caused by free radicals. It also refines the pores, tightens skin, reduces wrinkles , and age spots.

2 tbsp. mashed avocado

1 tsp. honey

1 tsp. almond oil

2 drops rose essential oil

Mix the avocado mashed in a bowl along with almond oil and honey until they create an even paste. Apply the paste to your face and let it sit to sit for fifteen minutes. Rinse off with warm water. To get the best results, use this mask at least once every week.

Face mask of avocado made from clay to treat oily skin

It controls the oiliness of the skin and deeply moisturizes the skin.

2 tbsp. mashed avocado

1 tbsp. natural clay

2 drops of essential oil tangerine to see if you're carrying it.

Make a paste of the avocado, then combine it with clay until they create an even paste. Apply it to your neck and face and let it sit for 15 minutes, then wash it off using lukewarm water.

Face mask made from avocados that is homemade and includes egg white

It regulates oiliness of the skin it hydrates the skin, slows the aging process and inflammation on the face.

1/2 avocado

1 egg white

1 tsp. freshly squeezed lemon juice

Mix the avocado that has been mashed together with egg whites as well as lemon juice into the bowl until they are an even paste. It is advised to apply the paste to your neck and face, keeping out the eye region. It should be left for 20 minutes, before washing it off with cool water. Make use of it every week.

Face mask of coconut oil made from home with lemon

Coconut oil is high in antioxidants, which include healthy acids like capric mystiric, caprylic and also lauric acids. It softens, smooths and smooth skin cells, eliminate dead cells, help heal acne, and moisturize skin. It boosts formation of collagen. It also fights free radicals and increases the elasticity of skin.

1 tbsp. coconut oil

2 tsp. raw honey

1/2 tsp. lemon juice

Mix these ingredients in a bowl. Apply the mixture to your face that is clean. Let it sit for 10 minutes and then wash it off using cool water. (Make sure to make use of coconut oil that is extra virgin to prevent the skin from irritation.)

Face mask made from coconut oil that contains banana and turmeric

This blend makes an excellent wrinkle and acne fighting mask. It reduces line wrinkles as well as fine wrinkles. and smooths and softens the skin. Additionally, it has anti-inflammatory and antiseptic and anti-bacterial properties.

1 tbsp. coconut oil

Half-ripe banana

A little bit of turmeric

Mash a half-ripe banana using a fork. Mix it with curcumin and the coconut oil until they make the consistency of a paste. Apply it to the skin and leave it for about

15 mins and then cleanse it using cool water.

Homemade oatmeal recipe that can be used to treat acne and eliminating dead cells

If you're seeking to treat acne, here's the recipe: boil oatmeal until it becomes soft and let it cool for 15 minutes . Then, after that, apply it to the area of concern and leave it sit on your skin for about 10 minutes. It will absorb and eliminate any excess oil and bacteria from your skin, and also exfoliate dead skin cells thus reducing acne. It's a great and effective method to treat your skin, and generally, it is very affordable and effective.

Home-made yogurt mask to treat acne

Because of the acidity of its nature, it kills numerous acne-causing bacteria, fungi and germs in the body. How can this be done?

Apply a thick, creamy yogurt on your face and leave it for 30 mins. After that cleanse your face by cleansing your face thoroughly. It is also possible to experiment using sugar, turmeric powder and sandalwood powder. You can make the paste and then apply it to your face over a period of 15 mins. Rinse off the paste with cold water.

Mask of yogurt made from homemade yogurt for anti-aging

To avoid wrinkles and to keep your skin young and youthful Try a facial pack made of 1erra. olive oil, and three tablespoons. yogurt. Apply it to the face and neck for 30 minutes , then repeat the process at least three times per week. It will begin to show results.

Another option to delay wrinkles is:

Mix avocado, banana and yogurt to form an emulsion and then apply it to your face for 30 minutes. Then cleanse your face.

Chapter 10: Science Of Aging Science Of Aging

Millions of years ago, life began with only one cell. Actually all anti-aging strategies originate from cells. We are just thousands upon millions of cell (37.2 trillion according to Smithsonian Magazine) that are connected by electromagnetic energy. Cells expand, divide, and then die at a staggering rate every second that we are alive from the time of conception until the time we pass away. Aging is the process when our body's cells begin changing or stop regenerate. To counteract the negative effects of aging, you must focus on our body's cellular levels.

Telomeres

If we are stressed out, we do not perform as efficiently. This can extend all the way to cells. Cellular stress could be caused by factors like toxins or inadequate nutrition, and these stressors can damage the DNA of the cells. Aging refers to the result of the accumulation of cells damaged that aren't getting replaced properly with healthy cells. The majority of cellular stress responses are caused by changes in cell reproduction and genes. The aging process is a reaction to the pathways in our body being degraded, in such a way that the messages to reproduce and renew between cells aren't getting through effectively. Imagine getting only half the directions to construct the bookcase. Cell reproduction is the same - cells must be provided with the proper signals and instructions or it won't multiply, divide or function as it should.

In all of our cells, there is DNA, the blueprint of our personal individuals. The DNA contains details about who we really are, which genetic characteristics we carry as well as what allergies and diseases we're susceptible to, and even the color of our eyes. It is the main reason for every physical characteristic we're born with. When cells divide the DNA inside it gets replicated in the cell that is to be replaced.

The last DNA chromosome is Telomeres. They function as tiny guidelines for the chromosones in the cell. If the copying of the DNA into cells is not completed, the telomeres may be cut , causing them to shrink and disappear a portion of the original data. Shortening of the telomeres is the main reason for ageing. Each time a cells divide, the shortening of telomeres occurs and the cell that is born will also be devoid of a part that originally contained the message that you have been given in your DNA. It's all about cutting down the length of telomeres for the longest time possible.

Your cells are always in the process of division, rejuvenating, healing and reproducing DNA to sustain your life. If your skin did not constantly renew , you'd have nothing remaining to substitute it when the cells that the cells you were born into die. In reality, it wouldn't be possible to have a baby because you were just a tiny cell prior to conception. Your telomeres keep shrinking and getting shorter because of this division , as well as those that aren't fully transmitting the instructions. When telomeres get too short, cells are unable to reproduce, which means that the tissue will eventually end up dying because new cells are not making themselves. There is no method to stop the telomeres from shortening , and consequently there is there is no way to stop the process of aging. However, we can slow the process of telomere lengthening, and thus slow down the process of aging.

There are a lot of telomeres that we have in our lifetime is variable. At conception , we can are blessed with up to fifteen thousand base pair of telomeres.By the time we're born, the number is at 10000. When we reach 5000 base pairs that is when the body starts to die from old age. The number of telomeres base pairs in your body can be the most reliable biological sign of the age discovered.It was initially believed that, through replication and division cells were immortal. However, during studies, Leonard Hayflick discovered that human cells are able to divide only about 60 times before they become too short to sustain the process, relying on the genes of both parents. This is called Hayflick's Limit. Hayflick Limit.

As recently as 200years ago, two scientists, Elizabeth Blackburn and Jack Szotak discovered an enzyme known as Telomerase. Telomerase extends telomeres by adding nucleotides at the end of the chromosome. it is present throughout every cell. In theory, if you filled every cell of the body with sufficient Telomerase you could reverse the process of aging. Blackburn and Szotak received the Nobel prize in the 'Physiology or Medicine' category for their work.

The main issue to this idea is that the quantity and amount of Telomerase as well as the effect it has on the different types of cells differs greatly. In some cells, Telomerase is more powerful than other cells. For instance, in cells of the ovary and testes there isn't any shortening of Telomeres. Your reproductive cells aren't aging! The reason is that these cells do not require replication. They're already in a half-formed form and need to be joined with the cells from the opposite sexe for division and reproduction to begin.

A study conducted at Harvard in 2010 examined mice genetically modified using Telomerase. The enzyme was able to maintain the tips of Telomeres as well as protected the end of their chromosomes against degradation. The mice aged reverse! The details of this amazing feat by reading The Harvard Gazette online. The exposure of human cells to the same enzyme can slow the aging process of cells and can even permit cells to reproduce in a new way.

This is a revolutionary idea in the world of aging. We've identified one enzyme that stops the process of aging and, in the right conditions, even cause its reverse. If you're interested in keeping your youthfulness to the maximum extent possible, the first goal you should set for yourself is to stop telomeres from shrinking. The goal is to slow down down telomere degeneration and encouraging maintaining the length of telomeres.

It is convenient that this breakthrough is already being used in supplements. Many of them are made from plants that aid in maintaining and repair the telomeres. They stimulate the telomerase that is already present in our bodies to slow the process of aging. Although they're not completely absolutely free, they must be thought of as one of the ways to protect yourself against the aging process.

Cell health and toxins

The Doctor Edward group, which is a specialist in anti-aging believes that the main causes of DNA changes that affect the telomeres are the effects of stress, toxins, and most importantly the passage of the passage of time. When you want to keep your cells youthful, they do are not just required to grow and reproduce properly, but also be able to do it quickly and efficiently enough to keep pace with ageing. Mitochondria are a tiny organelle that is found in the majority of cells. Its reproduction is crucial to the cell's youthfulness. The mitochondria inside cells produce energy in all forms physical and chemical. They transform nutrient chemicals into fuel that allows cells to perform. Without them , we wouldn't be able to accomplish anything. If it is a matter of energy production within our bodies, it is involving mitochondria.

One of the causes of aging is that mitochondrial efficiency decreases at the time we reach our 50s. Through our lives, our cells have to deal with wide range of substances, chemicals, and stressors that affect the cells. Toxins are absorbed by cells throughout our lives, and since they are within the cells, they be a part of the mitochondria inside our cells. As time passes, this interaction slows down the damage to mitochondria, and cells' capacity to use energy. Toxins are found in many varieties. Here are a few examples of how they can be found on junk foods. Alcohol, and pollution. The mitochondria and DNA through drinking alcohol and introducing contaminants to our systems.

If you don't live in a forest that is clean, has pure water, air and food that is organic, as well as not a lot of stress, it's likely that we'll be polluting our body to a certain degree. It's important to note that a lot of these toxins are easily avoided and it is possible to cut down on the intake of toxins from food as well as air and water.

Choose organic food whenever possible Eat whole foods Choose routes that have less pollution, or switch to water that is bottled - these are just some of the actions you can take to lessen the amount of the amount of toxins. In doing this, you can reduce the chance of the mitochondria being damaged and consequently to the cell's efficiency.Over time, this will reduce down the pace at which mitochondria's efficiency decreases.

The stress we've discussed is physical, but that's not one of the stressors that impacts our bodies.

The Other Types of Stress

Do you realize that stress from mental sources is also a factor in the reduction of telomeres? In our fast-paced world stress is the primary cause of the aging process. But stress can be multi-faceted when it comes to the process of aging. Stress can lead you to become older due to stress but it also keep you focused as well as make you less inclined to "give the fight" to get older. It's how you handle stress that's the key to remaining healthy, not the amount of stress is present in your life. Stress can affect telomeres through the increase of the amount of oxidative stress that can reduce the length, however only if you deal incorrectly.

Do not worry about it if you are experiencing plenty of stress! Everyone experiences anxiety throughout our lives. The constant avoiding of stress causes the body to be afraid of it, to the point that when it happens you feel the anxiety more strongly. People who are less stressed are those who accept the stress and don't get too worried about it. The main word in this case can be described as "perceived anxiety". It's not about whether or not you're stressed, which affects the telomeres of your body and your ageing rate, but how you deal with it or not.

Chapter 11: Chia Seeds

As you consider Chia seeds, you're probably thinking of the green and furry "pet" of which they were popular a long time ago. It was a time when the term "chia" was linked to the terms "cute" as well as "cuddly".

However, today there's a new story. The image of chia seeds has changed. Chia seeds that were previously considered to be an Aztec treasure that was forgotten for far too long but have returned to their splendor. When people mention chia today it is often a thought such as "energy", "protein" and, of the course "superfood".

Chia seeds look like tiny black sesame seeds. Do not buy red seeds since they're immature.

Essential Nutrients found in Chia Seeds

* Protein

* Dietary Fiber

* Omega 3

* Calcium

* Iron

* Manganese

* Phosphorus

* Potassium

* Antioxidants

Anti-Ageing Properties of Chia Seeds

Hydrates the skin Omega 3 promotes the production of healthy oils within your skin, which keep your skin soft and stops its flaking. You'll be pleased to learn Chia seeds contain eight times more omega 3 than salmon.

Reduce wrinkles Chia seeds can reduce the production of enzymes that degrade collagen. They also increase an Increase in elastin production making your skin youthful and firm.

Anti-inflammatory -- If you're experiencing irritation that you are unable to soothe, rubbing Chia gel to your face will soothe your skin.

Lip moisturizer apply chia gel it onto your lips, over the usual lip balm it will keep them longer hydrated and will not crack as easily.

Eliminate scarsChia gel is a great option to aid in removing marks and other imperfections. Apply the gel on the area of concern.

Keep your skin safe from cancerChia seeds safeguard your skin from negative effects of ultraviolet radiation.

Shiny hair If your hair is dull and dry Chia seeds can restore its shine, by encouraging oil production on your scalp.

Hair that is thicker Hair that is thicker Chia seeds can prevent hair loss.

Reduce the appearance of grey hair It's not a pleasant feeling to discover a new silver-colored hair appear. Chia seeds can slow down the development of grey hair and may even reveal the natural colour.

There's no more splitting endsChia oil serum helps heal split ends and stops further hair loss.

Enhances mental performance Omega 3 is known to aid in the development of neurological functions to prevent memory loss and enhance the brain's function.

aids digestion Get rid of constipation and bowel problems that aren't healthy. Chia seeds are high in phosphorus and fiber, you can include this into your diet and sleep more easily in the evening.

Cure sexual weakness The high levels of phosphorus in chia seed enable it to treat problems with weak sexual desire, for example sexual impotence and loss of libido.

Lose weight Chia seeds help will keep you fuller for longer. If you combine them with a proper fitness routine along with a balanced diet and routine, these supplements could help you shed a lot of weight , while also permitting you to work more and longer, and burn off more calories.

Controls blood sugar levelsChia seeds is more fiber-rich than half of a cup all-bran cereal. Other grains it is able to beat in terms of fiber content for dietary consumption are wheat, oats rice and corn. Due to its incredible high fiber levels, the grain regulates blood sugar extremely well.

Chia seeds are a great way to regulate sugar levels in your blood. that makes it an effective superfood for preventing the development of diabetes.

belly fat could be the result of insulin resistance. Chia seeds can reduce this problem by controlling blood sugar levels. This is what the high fiber content of chia seeds allows it to achieve.

Protects against cardiovascular disease This superfood has an extremely high amount of dietary fiber. This , along with calcium (which is also found in large amounts) are both essential nutrients that lower the risk of developing heart disease.

Increased energy levels Do you learn that chia seeds contain more protein than eggs? The superfood is famous for its energy-giving qualities. Additionally, when combined by itself, it makes an emulsion that provides the body with a superior level of water retention.

Repairs and builds muscleThe quantity of protein found in Chia seeds make it a top supplement to bulk up and building muscles.

fights depression Omega 3 is known as a depressive fighter Chia seeds are a great source of an incredible amount of omega 3 within them. It's quite amazing that a tiny seed has such amazing powers, isn't it?

Helps strengthen your bonesYour bones will stay strong. Chia seeds contain five times the amount of calcium as milk. This can prevent problems such as osteoporosis and hypocalcemia as well as osteopenia, fractured bones and fractures.

Beautiful teeth High levels of calcium and phosphorus allows the chia seeds to provide you with more healthy, beautiful teeth.

Aids in curing anemia Chia seeds contain three times the iron content of spinach. Consume chia seeds and be done with muscular weakness, body fatigue. Nights of sleeplessness, fatigue and trouble in concentration.

How to Make Use of Chia Seeds

Chia seeds may be consumed in their raw form or converted into gel using water added to. In either case there are plenty of recipes made of Chia seeds. They can be used to get healthy from your head to toes! Here are some fantastic recipes that are tasty and refreshing:

Chapter 12: Four Simple Things You Can Do to Keep Away Wrinkles

The most noticeable signs of aging can be seen on the face. Skin becomes wrinkled dry, dark, and stretched out. While various products for skin care promise reduction in dark spots and wrinkles however, no one is forever youthful. You can slow the process of aging but you cannot stop it. The issue with these products for skin care are that not all are healthy , and they aren't all efficient. Certain skin care products contain para-aminobenzoic acids, lead and formaldehyde, which are all harmful for cells and may even cause carcinogenesis. To stay away from the negative consequences of these products, explore these natural remedies for getting a more youthful-looking skin.

1. Guard your skin by shielding it from sun.

The ultraviolet rays released by the sun cause of serious skin cancers and cellular damage, so should be kept away from.

There are three methods to safeguard your skin from the harmful effects of sun's radiation. The first is to avoid taking a walk or being in the sunlight during the peak of UV rays' production. UV rays can be the most powerful between 10am and 4 pm, which is why it's better to stay home or reduce your exposure to sunlight during these hours. Also, make sure you use an umbrellas and hats with broad-brims before going out. Utilize UV-protected umbrellas to increase the protection you get. Wide-brimmed hats can be used to protect your face. The skin of your face is extremely thin and, therefore, extremely sensitive to the harmful effects of UV radiations. Skin darkening and wrinkles are just a few consequences of UV rays on your face. Also, make sure you wear protection clothing. Avoid wearing dark-colored clothing when you are out in the sun. Contrary to lighter-colored shirts that reflect only UV rays of the sun, dark shades tend to absorb UV rays which allows them to penetrate the skin.

2. Make sure you get the proper amount of sleep.

Cell renewal occurs during sleep hours and is most efficient when the body is in a relaxed state. Sleep deprivation can hinder the process of renewal and allow the cells that are senescent to remain. Skin cells are one of the most active cell types within the body, and they renew every couple of hours.This signifies that skin dead cells are always being removed from the body. If the process of cell renewal fails to take place and skin dead cells are left in your skin, it will get dry. Sleep deprivation can result in dark circles in the area of your eyes. The skin loses its natural glow when you do not get sufficient sleep.

If you're having trouble sleeping enough, there are some suggestions you can try:

Turn off the lights before you are sleeping. In addition to helping you sleep better and get better sleeping, shutting off the lights will reduce the risk of getting cancer. Contrary to what the majority of people think, UV rays are not only generated by the sun. Light bulbs can also release UV-rays when they are turned on. Therefore, it is recommended to switch off the lights in the evening when you are sleeping.

Avoid eating large meals prior to going to bed. The large meals can cause stomach pain and acid reflux while lying down. These issues can keep the ability to get a great night's sleep.

Avoid drinking a lot of water in the evening. In fact, drinking too much water prior to going to bed may affect your sleep patterns as the frequency of your urination rises. Drink plenty of fluids throughout the day, instead.

Relax and do not worry once you've settled into your mattress. Stress could keep you awake for the entire night and should be put away as you fall asleep.

3. Utilize organic scrubs and moisturizers, and exfoliates to improve your skin.

Extracts from some vegetables and fruits are a great scrub to use for your skin. Pick those that are high in antioxidants, such as orange, lemon, oatmeal and tea. You can mix sugar with tea or lemon juice to make facial scrub. Sugar crystals aid in removing dead skin cells, while the tea or juice provides antioxidants to your skin. Exfoliation doesn't just remove dead skin cells from the skin's surface and allows moisturizing and antioxidants to penetrate the skin more effectively.

It is also possible to moisturize your skin with no use of any most popular skin care products available there. Avocados and almond oil are great moisturizers because of the fats they contain. It is possible that you are worried because these are both high in fats, but there's nothing to worry about. Avocados and almonds contain healthy fats, including omega-3 fatty acids as well as HDL. Combine 3 tablespoons almond oil with one-half cup of avocado until it is smooth. Apply the cream to the face and neck for about 30 minutes , then wash off. It is possible to repeat this process every each night to get better results.

4. Keep your hands dry.

Your hands function as your identity card. Even if Botox treatments to your neck or face but you can't deny the signs of age that appear on the hands. Your hands are a source of an indication of your age, which is why it's best to shield your hands from the effects of aging as well. Apart from avoiding exposure toxic chemicals, you could use extracts of fruits to make an easy homemade moisturizer to your hands. You can mix orange , honey with lemon and uncooked rice to make the perfect hand scrub. Rice that has not been cooked can serve as an exfoliate, lemon, or orange can help lighten your skin, and keeps it glowing, and honey softens your skin.

Chapter 13: The Skin Care to Prevent Skin Aging

A balanced diet, along with good skincare routines can keep skin looking fresh and preventing premature ageing. Certain regimens for maintaining skin perform are more often out of habit than taking care of their skin. The skin's needs change as we get older. As you age the skin is more adept in repairing damaged skin cells, and the rate of cell regeneration is at its highest. As you age the skin gets dry and cells of the skin do not grow as fast as they used to. These changes must be addressed by implementing an overhaul of your skin care routine specifically designed for ageing skin.

For anti-aging, implementing with proper skin care in the early years is the best method to stop the aging of your skin. If you're already at the edge of getting older but are not enough time to start taking good care for your face. Nowadays, there are numerous skincare regimens you can follow to maintain your complexion youthful. Follow these steps to prevent wrinkles from appearing.

Washing

Wash using tepid water. Water that is too hot removes the skin's natural oils and leaves it dull and dry. Dry skin can be prone to cracks and flaking. The skin loses its elasticity as it ages , therefore it is recommended to keep your skin moisturized.

Cleanse your skin using the appropriate kind of facial wash. As you get older your skin may get dry. Make sure you use a facial wash that's also rich in moisturizers as well as other anti-aging ingredients.

Make use of circles and upward movements while washing. As your skin age becomes less elastic and can be prone to sagging. This is also caused by gravity. Cleanse your face using circular and upward motions to combat sagging skin. Making circular movements as you cleanse your face, you will promote proper blood circulation.

Do not wash more than twice a day. Too excessive washing can cause the skin to shed its oils. Wash your face once in the morning, and once at the end of the day before going to bed. Natural oils are essential to keep skin soft and dewy.

Don't rub-Pat your skin dry using a non-abrasive , soft towel. Avoid rubbing your skin since the skin is pulled which can cause wrinkles.

Creams and Serums

Moisturize, moisturise, and moisturize. This is possibly the most important skincare regimen you must follow to stop the aging process of your skin. The benefits of most moisturizers assist in maintaining its elasticity, and also hydrates the skin.

Sunblock- The sun's harmful rays are the most significant reason for premature aging on the face. If you're going out even if it's cold and dark, put sunblock to your body and face. Select a sunscreen that will shield you the skin from UVA and UVB radiation.

Night Cream- A night cream assists the skin heal itself as you rest. Pick a night cream that contains the ingredient retinol. Retinol is a potent component which boosts collagen production by stimulating repair of the skin and reduces dark spots on the skin. Night creams are designed for use while you rest.

Eye creamsEye creams work hand in hand along with the night-time creams. They must also contain Hyaluronic Acid and Retinol which help to keep moisture in the eyes. Be sure when applying eye cream that it is gentle on the eye area because they are the tiniest areas of skin on the face , and can be prone to wrinkles.

Spot correctors Spot correctors reduce darker spots that appear on your skin. Dark spots are an indication of ageing. The skin appears fragile and splotchy. Look for a moisturizer that contains hydroquinone. The ingredient fades dark spots that are caused by hyperpigmentation that occurs over time.

Makeup

Discover makeup specifically designed for your skin type - The anti-aging properties of makeup aren't only available in serums and creams. There are today makeup products and BB creams that have anti-aging ingredients , which promise less wrinkles in your skin. Certain face powders contain SPF.

Make sure you choose makeup that does not dry your skin. Dry skin can be an indication of aging. Find makeup that has moisturizing ingredients to nourish the skin.

Do not forget your lips. Lipsticks and lip balms that have the highest levels of moisturizing ingredients do more than make your lips look beautiful but also helps keep the lips's skin from becoming dry. Use a lip balm for times when you don't wish to be bothered by your lipstick.

Take off your makeup prior to going to bed . This routine for your skin can keep your skin looking healthy. All day long, pollution and other airborne bacteria have been absorbed by your makeup. By washing it off and removing it from your skin prior to hitting the toilet, you can prevent it from absorbing into the skin and cause damage over time. The inability to remove makeup can lead to breakouts of acne and pimples.

When selecting serums and creams make sure you select one designed specifically for your skin type. For instance, if you suffer from dry skin, select products that contain plenty of moisturizing ingredients. If you're prone to oily skin, choose products designed specifically for oily skin. When your skin appears sensitive, try the product on your skin prior to purchasing, or search for the products which have"good products for people with skin that is sensitive skin"on their labels.

Find products that are hypoallergenic and non-comedogenic-Hypoallergenic means it won't irritate your skin or trigger allergic reactions. Non-comedogenic which means it won't block pores.

Other important skin care routines for the face.

Weekly face masks Face masks are an excellent method for you to "deep clean"skin. Masks for face contain ingredients that stimulate cell renewal and shed dead skin cells and reveal new ones. They help to seal the skin with moisture so that it feels soft and firm.

Do it once or twice a month. A gentle scrub will remove dead skin cells and reveals fresher, smoother skin. Don't over exfoliate since this could cause skin damage and also. A complete body scrub performed by a professional may help you as they will penetrate areas in your body that you can't reach. Be sure to moisturize your skin or apply essential oils after you have exfoliated to lock in moisture.

Consult a dermatologist A dermatologist can provide the information you should know about the ageing skin. They will also offer treatments such as IPL or deep facial treatments, and other similar treatments.

Apply your moisturizer as soon as you've finished washing your face. after cleansing. If your the skin remains damp, apply your moisturizer since this is the ideal moment to allow it to penetrate the skin.

Wear appropriate clothing, a hat , and shades when you are outside in the sun. The sun's UV rays are the principal factor in premature aging.These products still provide some kind of UV protection, no matter how they are. Keep your shade in place when you are able.

The sun's rays can be at their most damaging from 9AM until 3PM. Stay inside whenever possible during these times. Even when it's cloudy the sun's rays could still penetrate through the dense clouds and cause damage to the skin.

Shower using lukewarm or cool water instead of a warm bath . The warm water causes the skin to dry out and flake. Dry skin appears aged and damaged. Make sure you keep the temperature of your bath at a minimum or after a bad day.

Chapter 14: Preventing Age from showing up on Your Face

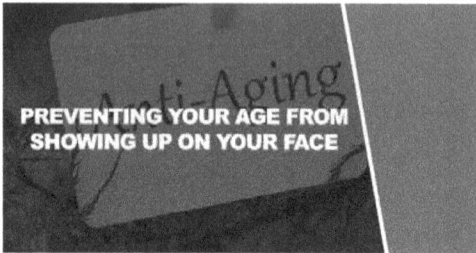

The skin is one of the most evident indicators of age. And if one asks someone else to estimate your age, it's your face that they will look at to form their estimation. This is why anti-aging skincare is among the best ways to look healthier and younger, making sure there aren't awkward moments where someone makes a mistake and thinks your sister as your daughter.

If you follow the right techniques It is possible to take the age of 25 to 25% off your appearance, perhaps more. You'll not only be more attractive but feel healthier too.

You can protect your skin by using the right nutrients

The most important aspect of anti-aging skincare is that of our diet. And the healthier our diet the more smooth and healthy our skin will become. This is logical when you think about the fact the fact that food supplies our body with the essential elements needed to maintain our skin as well as all other muscle and tissue within the body. You are the product of the food you eat and if you're looking to have healthy skin, it's best to follow to eat a balanced diet.

If you are thinking about how to age gracefully There are three primary items we should be incorporating into our diets - antioxidants fats and vitamins.

Antioxidants

First , the antioxidants in foods like fish and citrus fruits, can help to defend the skin cells (and all other cells) from oxidation and attack by free radicals. We've discussed this concept briefly in the past, but it is important to remind us that every cell in your body is constantly under attack by free radicals that harm the cell's walls when they come in contact with them.

There is enough of these abrasions and eventually, the microscopic injury is enlarged and your skin looks worn out and wrinkled. Even more concerning is that this damage may eventually make its way into your DNA, at which your cells are altered and appear damaged as they split. In the most extreme scenarios it could lead to the growth tumours that are cancerous. Antioxidants neutralize free radicals and ensure that they are fewer available to be able to attack the skin.

This will mean that skin cells are less under pressure and therefore appear healthier. In addition, this will to protect both the cells of your skin as well from cancer by reducing the risk of the DNA lining the cell walls becoming damaged or transformed.

There are many sources of antioxidants within your diet however the best way to ensure that you're getting plenty of them is to eat lots of vegetables and fruits that are usually packed with antioxidants.

Antioxidants include other things too, such as Resveratrol and CoQ10. You might recall from our nootropics section that they improve mitochondrial function. This is sense since damaging oxygen is a typical product of mitochondria, and it can result in damaging cells and the DNA .

Resveratrol is present in red grapes and red wine. It is thought to be the main reason that those living on the continent are less likely to suffer with heart diseases and other ailments!

Vitamins

Vitamins in turn, especially Vitamin A and E aid in the re-building of the skin. They are also an excellent way to help the body to heal wrinkles and marks. They help stimulate collagen production and other vital substances that provide the skin with its elasticity, and in general it will maintain your skin's appearance healthy and youthful. All of this comes from a diet that is rich in nutrients.

Fats

Essential fatty acids, in turn, give your skin oil that will keep it soft and stop it from getting dry, flaky. Omega 3 fatty acid can be a good source of oils for your skin, as well as an antioxidant source.

Saturated fats, in general, are an vital to your diet. They will assist keep your skin moisturized while also promoting your body to produce hormones which further assist in keeping your skin looking radiant.

Fats receive a lot of negative reviews in relation to health, however more recent studies suggest that we've turned them into blame-worthy individuals. Fat doesn't increase LDL (bad) cholesterol and it doesn't cause us to become fat. Fat is actually an essential element in our food!

And eating plenty of protein is equally important. Protein supplies the body with all the essential building blocks that it requires to make more tissues, which is the case for skin (not only muscles!).

The Best Diet to Look and feeling younger

With this all in mind, what's the best diet plan for looking and looking younger?

Actually, there's only one rule. It's to search for nutrition!

This also implies that you're better off staying away from these sugary carbs as well as processed foods such as chips cake, crisps and macaroni and chocolate,, and rice. These are all foods that increase blood sugar levels and reduce insulin sensitivity, increasing the risk of developing diabetes (which you're more at chance of developing as you grow older!). Additionally, these foods can increase your calories but don't provide any nutrients likely to improve your hair, skin and teeth, or nails. Why should you eat these foods?

Instead, look for fruit, vegetables such as salads, seafood, berries, meats and nuts as well as the delicious stuff that you will discover in the natural world. Smoothies are fantastic (although packed with sugar). Check out these superfoods! Did you have the knowledge that broth made from bones is brimming with collagen?

If you're in search of an organized diet plan that you can follow to help make this happen, there's plenty of options. The following tips will get you in the right direction:

*The Mediterranean Diet

*The Paleo Diet

*The Slow Carb Diet

And , guys, don't begin this process later when you begin to notice the signs of Aging increasing. Get started now , and you'll be in a position to keep the signs from happening. Prevention is better than treatment!

Have you eaten a lot, or a Little?

There's a second question whether you should take in a lot of food or only eat a few bites?

This is among the top questions you can consider when you are looking younger. your goal in reality!

On the other side, there's an ideology which suggests that you should eat only a small amount. This is known as 'Calorie Restriction' and is exactly as it states on the box. The idea behind this is that by limiting calories, you'll be able to decrease the rate of getting older and stay younger for longer.

How do you accomplish this? According to some proponents eating less calories means mitochondria function less, and therefore produce less free radicals. Your body has to depend on ketones, and is extremely efficient at storing energy (eating low-carb diets may have the same impact, as could intermittent fasting). Research suggests that mice that are on low-calorie diets can increase their life span by up to 30%. There many enthusiastic individuals who are trying this method currently. Can it be effective for humans? It's too early to say.

With all that being said there are some real negatives of this method as well. One of them is that it increases the risk of malnutrition. Although a healthy diet should not cause malnutrition, it's obviously much more difficult to get all the nutrients you require from your body when eating a small amount of calories.

It's also not feasible for the majority of us, and isn't the most enjoyable.

There's a second argument that suggests being a little puppy-fat will make your appearance appear younger as you get older. As we get older our skin thins and we begin to have less subcutaneous fat (fat that is stored underneath your skin). This means that we begin to appear more attractive. Consider comparing a thin woman to a lady who is eating a lot however, and you'll see that the former looks younger due to their skin being smoothed due to the fat layer below.

In contrast, they'll usually have more color and be healthier. Women claim that when they enter their 60s and 50s and 60s, they must decide between 'face' or 'body'.

What can you do? That's up to you, however, make sure that no matter what method you decide to adopt, you're focusing on nutrition within your food!

Skin Care to Prevent Aging

The treatment of anti-aging skin can also be a matter of lifestyle and the way we treat our bodies will show by the way our skin appears. While sun exposure will make us appear healthy and bronzed in the short-term but over time, it can result in damaged skin cells, which will cause more wrinkles in our older years. This could lead to wrinkles and age spots, as well as other problems due to the UV radiation that the sun emit damage to cells and trigger mutations. Shade and sunblock can reduce this in a significant way.

It's also important to ensure that we're sleeping well. One reason to this is because our sleep is the time that our bodies repair the damage that has been caused to our bodies during the day, and can help rejuvenate our skin in this way. One method by that this happens is through production of the growth hormone also known as HGH that is a hormone that stimulates anabolism within the body, making it heal wounds, build muscles, replace damaged cells, and promote growth in bones and muscles (though bones do not grow as puberty approaches and the growth plates stop growing). Along with sleep, another method of encouraging the natural growth hormone production (synthetic growth hormone) is to use it frequently by bodybuilders and famous people however it is banned in the majority of countries and states, and extremely expensive in the ones are not - it can also cause a number of negative adverse effects, some of which can be dangerous) is to work out and take hot showers as both can cause an anabolic process.

HGH is possibly the closest thing to a magic potion of youth at the moment, so any action you can take to increase it naturally certainly be to be encouraged.

Creams and other Products

The most obvious part of skincare is using anti-aging creams and other products. They work in a variety of ways, both shielding your skin from damage from UV rays and other environmental elements, as well as providing your skin with vital antioxidants and nutrients applied to the skin. They also help to hydrate your skin and even tighten it in certain situations to offer instant advantages.

It is important to ensure that you adhere to a schedule and apply your creams to your face each morning and at the evening before going to going to bed. This should start with an exfoliating cream or wash to remove the dead cells of your skin (that might interfere with the mechanism of moisturizing creams and the nutrients). Exfoliating may also make wrinkles appear less noticeable because it brings your skin to the same amount and will give your skin an overall healthy glow (dead skin appears slightly greyer). This will instantly help you look and appear younger.

(Another option to have more glow is to get some natural tan. The best method to achieve this without risking sun damage is to use self-tanning lotion. This isn't fake , it's an ingredient that increases melanin production naturally and give you a more radiant appearance. This could help you avoid the grey, washed-out appearance that's often commonly associated with old age.)

Following this, you must apply a cream that is protective like Protect and Perfect for No. 7, which protects your skin from sun's UV-rays as well as the effects of oxidative. Then, a moisturizing moisturizer should be applied that must contain vitamin A as well as E both of which are essential in the repair of skin and collagen. These will aid in keeping the skin plump and elastic (it could be described as nature's Botox'). Certain creams contain collagen however there is some doubt about whether they is able to penetrate deep enough into the lower layers of the skin to provide any benefits. Some products, like Bio Oil claim to contain carriers and other methods to overcome this issue. Check your backside of package for any moisturizer, and look out for items such as biotin (vitamin B7) and retinol. Also, look for Green Tea Extract, CoQ10 etc. Beware of the claims of big names however, and make sure to read reviews before committing your money you've earned. There are many alternatives to choose from, such as applying hemorrhoid cream to the eyes to improve skin tightness and eliminate crow's feet. If you're looking to play with this then go for it however for the most part, there's no need to overspend and any moisturizer that is healthy (ideally organic, like a deep-sea mud) can do the trick.

The moisturizing ingredient will aid in hydrating the skin and make it more subtle and flexible. When applying the creams, apply circular motions using finger pads to rub your skin and increase blood flow to the skin that will provide the skin with more essential nutrients, and help keep the complexion more uniform. Utilize concentric circles as you move towards the middle of the face. It's also extremely comfortable and helps to keep your skin looking subtle and soft.

Whatever you pick be sure that you're using something that will exfoliate, something that will protect and to revitalize and moisturise.

Chapter 15: Skin Care Products.

Each year, billions of dollars go into skincare products. The public is often bombarded with advertisements for various products that are available. We're left to wonder which one is the best choice for us. In this article, we are going to review the most effective skin care products your skin needs. Because of a better knowledge of how skin ages, contemporary skincare products are more efficient. They are made up of multiple ingredients which are designed to conceal wrinkles and wrinkles on the face.

Moisturizer/hydrating cream

As we age, our skin deteriorates and often we experience more dry feeling. The skin loses its ability to retain moisture for prolonged periods. Dryness increases, which leads to dry skin and wrinkles across the body. Moisturizing creams and moisturizers are a great way of making sure your skin looks beautiful along with other treatments, primarily nutrition and supplements that moisturize by nourishing the inside, if you want your skin to look younger, it needs to be well-hydrated. Dry skin looks older.You might not have noticed this during your younger years, but as you age you'll be looking to use the best moisturizer.

They are specifically designed anti-aging moisturizers that are designed to counter the effects of age. They're intended to decrease wrinkles and increase elasticity. Applying moisturizers to your skin is an absolute must when you want to reverse the signs of aging skin. What moisturizing creams do is help to smooth out the wrinkle lines that are already visible so that they are less noticeable and also reduce their appearance when you apply new wrinkles. To select the most effective moisturizing cream, we have be aware of the ingredients. It should contain vitamin E Vitamin C, retinol, Vitamin B5 and Alpha-hydroxy acids as well as ferulic acid. Olive oil is an essential ingredient in moisturizing products. It isn't possible to incorporate all the ingredients listed above in one product but the more , the more effective. These are essential vitamins that are required by our skin. Another aspect to be considered is that the moisturizer can have a an extended effect over the day.

Sunscreen

Sunscreens protect us from sun's rays. The sun's UV ultraviolet rays are extremely damaging for the skin. After a brief time in the sun, without sunscreen, you damage your skin and get older more quickly. There's lots of studies that show that the possibility of developing skin cancer when they are on the hot sun for extended durations. Sunscreen is able to absorb these harmful UV rays and creating an insulator against them on the face. Don't go outside in sunlight and not apply sunscreen.

With all the sunscreens available on the market it is possible to be overwhelmed in deciding which one is the most effective.

This is exacerbated due to the fact that there is inconsistent information about the efficacy of the products. Some guidelines to take into consideration prior to purchasing sunscreen include:

* Broad spectrum sunscreens that have values over 15 are recommended.

They are believed to be superior to sprays, powders or lotions. This is due to the fact that the theory is that creams protect the skin more effectively. Sprays and powders can be breathed into the body, which can be harmful.

* The sunscreen must be water resistant to provide the greatest protection. Sunscreens that are easily removed with sweat can expose you to.

*If you're a parent with children choose a sunscreen suitable for the skin of your children.

Find out what kind of skin and the best sunscreen for it. Are you prone to dry or oily skin? Is your skin sensitive? Are you suffering from some skin problem, such as acne or Psoriasis?

* Make sure that you are aware of the contents and make sure you are safe to use them on your face. You may want to consult the advice of a dermatologist for the right sunscreen for you in case your skin is suffering from medical issues. The most known toxic ingredients in sunscreens are diethanolamine, imidazolidinyland polyethylene glycol, as well as the phthalates.

The sun's rays cause ageing of the skin. If you are looking to keep your youthful appearance ensure that you wear sunscreen prior to going out in the sunlight.

Sunscreen and moisturizer are two essential anti-aging products. It is essential to apply these products regularly to see improvement on your skin. When we have completed our 30 days, you will see significant changes to your skin.

Chapter 16: Sensory Function (Vision and Hearing Smell, Taste and Touch)

Our senses gather information from our environment, and the information they receive including sound, light taste, smell and even touch - is transmitted through neuronal signals for the brain. The brain interprets the sensations.

As you age, you gain wisdom However, the reality is that as you age, you actually see the world differently due to the fact that your senses are affected. The way you perceive and hear, feel, feel, and smell fades as the years go and go by. These changes may affect the our quality of life. It can happen that the activities are less enjoyable and communications become more complicated and people may start feeling isolated. As the information gathered from the surroundings becomes less clear, the minimum amount of stimulation needed to take in any feeling (called"the threshold) is increased. This implies that the threshold gets more intense as we age.

While hearing and sight are the two most commonly affected by aging, any of the senses are affected. The use of equipment and other devices is often introduced to enhance sensory experience and improve the quality of life for those who are older (hearing aids, glasses, for instance) however, other efforts can be taken to stop the aging process of sensory perception, or to help the natural changes. Let's examine each sense each in turn, and discuss the methods that can aid.

Vision

The brain processes light through the eye as it moves through the cornea. It then travels through the pupil and is interpretable through the brain. This is the reason why the pupil grows and shrinks in order to control the quantity of light that passes through the eye. When light is absorbed the lens, the eye's inner part focuses the light to the retina, which converts it into signals that send to the brain through the optic nerve.

With age our pupils shrink in size. actually they shrink by approximately 2/3 as we age from 20 to 60. Also, they react in different ways to dark and bright light and the cornea is less sensitive, which makes injuries to the eye less apparent. Additionally lenses of eyes gets clouded in color, becomes yellow, and less flexible, and the muscles of the eye are less flexible and move more freely. The floaters can also block your vision. As you age, these particles known as vitreous, float in the eye. While they aren't blinding, they are annoying. The weaker eye muscles can restrict peripheral vision, which causes the fields of vision to shrink. This all contributes to the diminishing of vision. Focusing becomes harder, glare becoming less tolerated, and seeing in darkness decreased drastically. This can make driving at night, or sitting out in the bright light of the afternoon, difficult on the eyes.

It becomes harder to distinguish between cool and neutral shades like greens and blues. This is the reason why bright and warm colors can enhance vision. It's recommended to illuminate rooms at night by using an orange light instead of white light.

Furthermore, eyes that are aging create less tears which leads to dry eyes. These are more prone to infection, inflammation and cornea scarring. Eye problems, such as macular degeneration and glaucoma or cataracts, may also develop.

Eye exercises can help improve vision because of eyestrain and greater sensitivity to light also blurred and distorted eyes. Through strengthening the muscles around the eyes, eye focus and movement are improved. The brain's visual center is activated by a series of exercises to control eye muscles. For instance, covering each eye individually and focusing on different objects, or focusing on one thing or following a particular visual pattern. The natural patterns vary in accordance with the current eyesight problem and the patient's age.

Essential oils may help in the fight against macular degeneration. Take a look at this study released in Molecular Vision, which examined the effects of a mix with zinc oxide as well as Rosemary oil on retina damage caused by light.

Study 5 Vision

"Zinc oxide reduces the risk of the loss of visual cells in rodents exposed to intense light. It is also known to reduce the rate of the progression of disease in the advanced stages of macular degeneration caused by age. Our objective was to assess the effectiveness of zinc oxide when combined with well-established and novel antioxidants in a animal model of retinal oxidative damage...In the rat model for acute retinal light-induced damage, zinc oxide in conjunction along with the detergent extract from Rosemary oil or Rosemary powder has more efficacy than treatments with any component on its own and considerably more efficient than an AREDS mix with a similar dose of zinc oxide. Oxidative stress from light-induced in animals models of retinal degeneration could be an effective preclinical model for evaluating novel antioxidants as well as for testing therapeutic strategies that can slow the progression of eye diseases."

In the study , one group of rats were subjected to treatment with zinc oxide or Rosemary extract in separate doses and then under intense sunlight for between 4 and 24 hours. Another group was treated with the combination consisting of zinc oxide with rosemary oil, and the third group received an antioxidant mineral mix that contained zinc oxide. After two weeks of intensive light therapy, the vision cell survival of rats was assessed and the results revealed that the combination of zinc and Rosemary boosted visual cell survival and also reduced the expression levels of stress markers. The results suggest that oils with essential components, particularly Rosemary can be useful supplementation in treatments for visual therapy and may help prevent ocular degeneration and diseases.

Essential Oil Protocols

Eyesight loss

Description:

Presbyopia (failing eyesight) is a natural occurrence with age because the elasticity of the lens of the eye is diminished. Presbyopia can manifest in different forms, such as cataracts that cause cloudy or foggy vision that results from conditions such as eye surgery, diabetes trauma, congenital defects or radiation-related - the glaucoma condition, where drainage of the eye fluid is hindered, causing damage to the optic nerve. This can result in loss of vision - retinal detachment blurred vision due to the retina's separation from tissues beneath it; could be caused by injury or inflammation, as well as conditions like diabetes, the uveitis/irititis condition - inflammation or irritation of the uvea or the iris that is caused by autoimmune disorders or infections - and macular degeneration which blurs the central vision zone caused by the aging process.

Application:

To help regenerate, put 1 or 2 drops of your preferred oil on your fingertips (Anti-Aging Blend Frankincense or Helichrysum can be all suggested) and rub the oil all over the eye socket, but do not put it directly into the eye. Repeat this three times per day. Also, dilute your selected oil by using a carrier oil, and massage it into the reflex points on the feet. Eye problems that result from infections (like iritis and uveitis) may benefit from an Detoxification Cleanse, or from an Anti-infectant program.

Recommended oils:

Ylang Ylang, Sandalwood, Rosemary, Lemongrass, Lavender, Helichrysum, Frankincense, Cypress and Anti-Aging Blend

Other Natural Methods of Treatment:

Think about essential oils-based products such as The Detoxification Blend, the GI Cleansing Formula and the Probiotic Defense Formula. Ginkgo biloba boosts the circulation of the eye, preventing macular degeneration as well as glaucoma. It can also help improve the vision. Every day , take a 120 mg capsule, divided into 3 doses.

Hearing

The ears serve two purposes They help maintain body equilibrium and, of course they also hear. Balance is controlled through tiny hairs and the fluids in the ear's inner part that are sent via an auditory nerve, which connects to brain, aiding in maintaining equilibrium. Hearing happens when sound vibrations reach the inner ear through the eardrum. After that, the inner ear converts the vibrations to nerve signals, which are sent to the brain through the auditory nerve.

The aging process alters the structure that make up the inner ear. This can which results in decreased function and lessening the capacity of the ear to comprehend sounds and maintain the balance. Hearing loss is often affecting both ears, and is especially relevant for high-frequency sounds , and distinguishing between distinct sounds. Background noise can also affect the ability to hear and other ailments - such as tinnitus can create unusual sounds, like rings. This can result from hearing loss or earwax accumulation.

Essential Oil Protocols

Hearing Loss

Description:

Hearing loss occurs when one or both ears not hear normally and, in turn, not be able to understand certain frequencies, words or background noise. Hearing loss is a natural process with age and can be caused by the loss of hearing due to conductive causes (eardrum damaged due to accumulation of fluids, wax and infections) and sensorsineural loss of hearing (nerve ends inside the ear have stopped responding properly due to aging, disease or medications) as well as hearing loss that is congenital (hearing hearing loss in the earliest years of life due to the genetic abnormality or infection).

Application:

Blend 4 drops of the Calming Blend with Grounding Blend. Apply it topically on in the front part of your ears, over the fleshy rim, along the earlobe, as well as through the Eustachian tubes that run under and behind the ears, and then behind the line of jaw. Do this 10 times. Apply 4 drops of Helichrysum by the same way and repeat five times. Mix 2 drops in White Fir, and Lavender and apply using the same way. Repeat five times. Apply 3 drops of Geranium using the same method and repeat three times. Inhale and cup. Repeat the process 3 times per week for 6-8 weeks.

Recommended oils:

White Fir, Lavender, Helichrysum, Geranium, Fennel, Eucalyptus, Grounding Blend, and Relaxing Blend

Other Natural Methods of Treatment:

Ginkgo biloba boosts blood circulation and may help those suffering from hearing loss. Every day , take a 120-mg capsule , broken into 3 doses.

Tinnitus

Description:

Tinnitus is when a loud sound (ringing or whistling or buzzing) can be heard in the ear, with moderate or insufferable effects. Tinnitus is a sign that usually is a sign of a health issue that could be a sign of an ear infection or allergy fluids, physical injury in the eardrum (loud sounds) or wax buildup. It may cause ear pain due to age or certain medication.

Application:

Mix 1 drop each from Basil with Frankincense and apply the mixture topically over the ear, and along the jaw line, all the way to the chin. Repeat the process several times and adhere to the procedure every 1-4 hours, or until sound stops.

Recommended oils:

Rosemary and Peppermint Lavender, Helichrysum, Geranium, Frankincense, Cypress, and Basil

Other Natural Methods of Treatment:

Think about essential oil-based products such as GI Cleansing Formula or Probiotic Defense Formula. Ginkgo biloba increases blood circulation, and can aid people suffering from hearing loss. Each day, take a 120-mg capsule divided into a couple of doses.

Vertigo

Description:

Vertigo is a condition that occurs because the body's balance is unable to function properly, usually due to a lack of connection between the vestibular organ in the inner ear as well as the brain.

Vertigo causes your surroundings to appear like they're in motion, causing imbalance and nausea.The problem could also result from injuries to the body, swelling or chemical imbalances.

Application:

To help prevent vertigo, dilute your selected oil in the same way (Ginger is recommended) by using a carrier oil , and apply the oil topically on the affected area.You may also put some drops inside capsules and consume in a pill. To ease an attack, put a couple of drops of your oil of choice (Frankincense is recommended) under your tongue when you feel a sense of instability comes over your. Repeat after 30 minutes.

Oils to be recommended:

Ylang Ylang, Thyme, Rosemary, Roman Chamomile, Peppermint Lavender, Helichrysum, Ginger, Geranium, Frankincense, and Basil

Other Natural Methods of Treatment:

Think about essential oil-based products such as for instance the Basic Vitality Supplement (LLV). If you're feeling dizzy, do a deep breathing exercise to relax the nervous system and supply an oxygen supply to your brain. lay down or sit comfortably, place your hands on your abdomen, with the thumb on the opposite hand on one nostril. close your mouth and inhale slowly until your lung is full of air. Hold the breath for a few seconds and then exhale slowly. Repeat 10 times and remain in a calm state for five minutes until you feel less dizzy.

Taste and Smell

The senses of smell and taste are synergistic senses since odors usually directly affect your sense of tasting. The nerve endings that line the upper nasal lining are the place where smell starts and tastes are defined by the more than 9000 taste buds that distinguish the difference between sweet, salty, acidic, or bitter taste. Together, they are used to recognize hazards, like gas, smoke decay, or spoilage.

As you age , your taste buds diminish in size They lose their mass in addition to their capability to discern the differences between four tastes decreases. Additionally there is less saliva produced, which could cause dry mouth. It can also affect the taste.

The smell may also decrease because of the nose's reduction in nerve endings, along with the production of less mucus. Because of this, the lack of nerve endings, and the decrease in mucus odor, the smells aren't retained in the nose for sufficiently long to allow them to be able to detect. Nasal polyps can also interfere with smell, and could cause breathing difficulties.

A few factors that affect the speed that you lose the senses are smoking, certain illnesses and exposure to pollution and other harmful air particles. If smell and taste disappear, the chance of danger rises, because our sense of smell typically draws our attention to hazardous situations, like burning or toxic gases. In addition, appetite can be decreased, because the taste buds aren't working properly there isn't any pleasure to be gained from food.

There are a few natural remedies which can help to prevent the loss of smell and taste. It is possible to alter the food you prepare to include specific spices that can trigger taste, for example, Ginger or Garlic. You may also want to speak with your doctor when you have issues that are related to a specific medication you've been given.

Essential oils can stimulate flavor and smell by stimulating taste and smell in these ways.

Essential Oil Protocols

Dry Mouth

Description:

Bad breath and dry mouth (halitosis) is often due to health issues or poor oral hygiene or the aging process. Lifestyle choices that are unhealthy can cause the issue, as do the food you consume.

Application:

Two drops of your preferred oil on your tongue.

Recommended oils:

Wintergreen, Peppermint, Fennel and Digestive Blend

Other Natural Methods of Treatment:

Take a look at essential oil-based items, such as Peppermint Beadlets. Fennel is also a great remedy for bad breath and dry mouth by chewing a teaspoon of Fennel seeds slowly, as it can stimulate saliva production.

The loss of smell (Anosmia)

Description:

The loss of smell, also known as anosmia can be an ongoing or temporary condition in which the physical pathways that connect the nasal passages to the olfactory cells have been blocked or the nerve pathways in the brain aren't functioning. It can also influence taste as both are linked. Anosmia is caused by sinus congestion and nasal polyps. Other causes include allergies, sinus congestion and toxic chemicals, medicines or drugs, imbalances in nutritional and hormonal levels and certain diseases like Alzheimer's, Parkinson's or multiple sclerosis.

Application:

*Clear nasal obstructions by diffusing or apply the cupping method by inhaling the Respiratory Blend. You can dilute the essential oil according to (Rosemary, Basil, and Tea Tree are suggested) and apply it to the sinuses, around the eyebrows and the nose.

*Stimulate the olfactory system by inhaling Repiratory Blends or Peppermint regularly and often using the cupping technique.

Oils to be recommended:

Rosemary Respiratory Blend Peppermint Tea Tree Lime and Basil

Other Natural Methods of Treatment:

Think about GI Cleansing Formula/Probiotic Defense Formula, or Cellular Complex. Warm up a tablespoon. from castor oil by heating it in the microwave couple of seconds. Place one drop into each nostril two times every day, in the morning and at evening.

Nasal Polyps

Description:

A polyp is generally benign, though sometimes it is a protuberance that is cancerous or pre-cancerous mucus membrane. It can be directly connected or have a lengthy stock that connects them to their body. They typically occur on the colon, nasal passages, cervix and the urinary tract. The symptoms include bleeding that is abnormal (cervical polyps) or breathing issues (nasal polyps).

Application:

Nasal polyp - put 3 to 4 drops of your preferred essential oil (Frankincense and Tea Tree are both suggested) using a Q-tip, then apply it to your nose's bridge, and under the tongue. You can also consume it internally, in capsules, for up to two times a daily.

Other polyps - put three drops of Frankincense on the tongue or as a capsule.

Recommended oils:

Peppermint Oregano oregano, tea Tree, Lemon, Lavender, Grounding Blend, Frankincense, Cleansing Blend and Basil

Other Natural Methods of Treatment:

Eliminate toxic substances by eating cayenne peppers as well as drinking hot tea in the heat. The two will trigger sweating and rid your body of toxins that can affect the growth of polyps.

Touch (Pain and Vibration)

The nerves in joints, tendons muscles, skin and internal organs that transmit signals to the brain concerning the temperature, vibration and pressure, as well as pain and the location in the physique. Although the information could be in the subconscious, there are times when the information can trigger a sharp sensations, as the brain recognizes the type and strength of the touching.

As you age , your senses could change or decrease due to nerve end-to-end damaged, decreased blood flow to the brain, or spinal cord injury. As such, many of the functions that are associated with the brain - like nerve damage and circulation may also cause loss of the sense of. Also, health issues could cause changes in sensation, and so can an absence of nutrients.

If the sense of the touch is diminished, there is a higher chance of injury from temperature, specifically in relation to hypothermia, burns, or frostbite. Also, the individual could be unaware of pressure ulcers, other painful or injuries because of the decrease in sensitivities. On the other side in the range, certain people develop an abnormal sensitivity any touch to the skin as a result of the skin's thinness due to age.

Some guidelines for staying secure include dressing appropriately for the weather, keeping track of how hot the water is in order to prevent burns, and examining yourself for any injuries.

Essential Oil Protocols

Heat Exhaustion/Heat Stroke

Description:

The process of exhaustion causes heat when the body's capacity for cooling itself becomes not sufficient to the demands of physical exertion due to extreme heat or humid conditions sweating, dehydration, or both. The symptoms include an increasing temperature, a the appearance of a flushed face, weakness and disorientation. Heat stroke occurs if the temperature rises above 104 F. Seek medical attention, as symptoms of heat stroke also include increased heart rate, vomiting, diarrhea, convulsions/seizures, unconsciousness, and flushed color in other body parts.

Application:

Apply a couple drops of peppermint to an ice-cold, damp cloth and apply it on the forehead. For application on the skin Apply 3 to 4 drops of Peppermint onto the neck, chest and the neck's back as well as the soles of your feet. Utilize the cup and inhale method, and if the body temperature increases dramatically, apply an ice bath.

Recommended oils:

Lavender and Peppermint

Other Natural Methods of Treatment:

In the first place, take the person to a shaded and cool place, then rehydrate them with cool drinks (avoid drinking carbonated alcohol and carbonated beverages) and put them in a relaxed place.

Sensory Processing Disorder

Description:

Sensory Processing Disorder (SPD) is a condition that occurs when the sensory information is not processed properly and causes overreactions or under reaction to specific sensory experiences, such as sensitivity to light, the touch of certain textures or odors or even displays of extreme distress and fear and tantrums over minor incidents and not interfacing with others, appearing uncoordinated or needing sensory stimulation prior to going to sleep. The cause for this condition is unclear.

Application:

The oil to be diluted according to (a mixture comprising 18 drops Vetiver 10 drops Lavender 10 drops Ylang Ylang and 7 drops Frankincense and 5 drops Clary Sage, 3 drops Marjoram and 12 drops fractionated coconut oil an oil roller bottle is recommended for use with only a single roll of the mix) using an oil carrier and apply it topically on the soles of feet as well as the neck's back and to the suboccipital triangle.

Conclusion

I'm sure by now you're as thrilled about the ways that a healthy raw diet will aid you to combat the signs of aging as I am.The details in this book will aid you in starting an entirely new way of living - since raw veganism isn't just an eating plan, it's an ideal lifestyle choice that can completely change your body from the inside out.

If you stop for a moment to consider the many chemical additives in food and the chemicals we put into and on our bodies, there's no wonder that many of us are getting older more quickly than we were able to.Life can be extended however lives are artificially extended by drugs or surgeries.More and more are suffering from chronic diseases such as cancer and heart disease.Most people read their the food labels and, when we do, we remind ourselves that food makers aren't allowed to use substances into our food if they were not healthy.